Good Raw Food Recipes

Good

Raw Food

Recipes

Delicious Raw and Living Food

for Energy and Wellness

Judy Barber

RETHINK PRESS

First Published in Great Britain 2012 by RethinkPress.com

Ink sketches, cover photo and cover art – Amelia Parisian
Pencil drawings – Rich Simpson
Photos – Judy Barber

The recipes and information in *Good Raw Food Recipes* are provided by the author for informational and educational purposes only. The views expressed are purely the author's own views and opinions of certain issues that pertain to health and nutrition and are based on her own experiences. Use of the material set forth in the following pages is at the reader's discretion and is his or her sole responsibility. Questions about food, diet, nutrition, natural remedies and holistic health should be directed to a professional healthcare practitioner.

This book is for everyone who helped me, and for those who create delicious, nourishing food; food that promotes vitality for you, your family and your friends, for making your unique positive contributions in life.

Contents

Introduction

Why Raw Food?

Raw food from plants is fresh and full of life. It is the no-cook food that can provide reliable energy all day and help you look and feel good. A tiny sprouting seed has the potential to grow into a big plant, and that potential for life nourishes and energises us. Raw food is delicious, and many more people are finding it improves their enjoyment of life and their ability to heal.

Raw food is a new world to explore. Here are simple but novel ways with soups, salads, tasty savoury dishes, satisfying sauces and dressings, and sweet raw treats.

In a nutshell:

- Cooking destroys some of the nutrition in food. People spend money on food and then destroy some of its value before eating it.
- Food enzymes start being destroyed at around 46° Centigrade/115° Fahrenheit. Up to a point our bodies recycle and create enzymes. This happens less with age and then enzymes in fresh food become much more important.
- Raw vegetables provide plenty of enzymes and important nutrients that support us in leading healthy energetic lives.
- Our bodies have living electrical balances of alkaline/acid biochemistry. Like cars, if we have flat batteries we cannot get far, so we need to top them up with raw and living food. Most conventional diets are far too acidic. Disease can be initiated or made worse in acidic conditions. White flour, sugar, meat and milk are some of the most acidic culprits.

❧ Uncooked food from plants can be healing and invigorating, something which is being discovered by more and more people, including me.

What is Raw and Living Food?

This is raw vegan food from plants. It includes sprouts and freshly picked tray greens that are still alive and growing when you eat them, hence *Raw and **Living***.

Sprouts and tray greens, and soaked seeds and nuts, have far more enzymes and vastly increased nutrition compared with adult plants. Many feel they are essential to a raw food way of eating.

My Interest in Raw Food

I tumbled into the world of raw food at a time when I was tired and feeling flat. Looking back, I had become bored. My passion for creating delicious meals was, unusually for me, absent.

When I changed my way of eating, I cheered up and found a spring in my step very quickly. Life in general improved, my appetite picked up and my joy in food returned. Having whole new vistas of food was, and still is, enjoyable and exciting. I still love creating and eating raw food meals. There is the intrigue of creating comfortably familiar dishes, and the scary pleasure of inventing afresh from the tastes and textures of raw plants.

Raw and living vegan food has possibilities that are very different from cooked food. Countless meals can be made with so much creaminess, crunch, smoothness, juiciness, variety and exquisite mixtures of tastes that the diners are too absorbed in the joys of eating to consider nutrition or how different this may be from their accustomed fare.

Why Have I Written *Good Raw Food Recipes?*

Since the beginning of 2008 I have been eating mainly raw food and have learned a huge amount from some who have been eating and teaching about raw and living food for many years, in person from Dr Brian

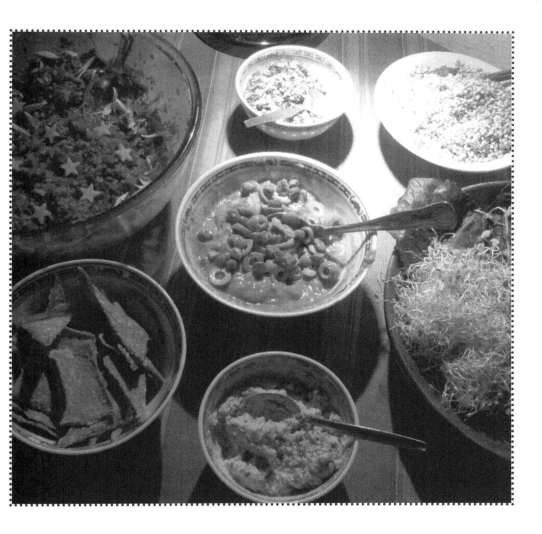

Dinner Chez Judy: Home grown greens and sprouts, Avocado and
Red Pepper Salsa, Beetroot Salad with carrot stars, Cucumber
Relish and dehydrated crackers

Clement, Dr Anna Maria Clement, Viktoras Kulvinskas, Dr Gabriel Cousens and Shakti Cousens.

I want to pass on what I know.

If you want to read about my own food story, you will find it at the end of the book.

Good tastes and textures, whether in complex gourmet dishes or in simple meals, keep me going. Most of my meals at home are 80-100% raw and living vegan. When under the weather, I go 100% raw, but when I am well, active and out and about, I have some cooked foods and rare sweet treats.

Sometimes in social situations I choose to go along with what is served. If I had to heal a serious illness, health condition or injury, I would, however, be totally strict. I have witnessed how fast people can heal themselves this way.

Raw food is my default habit. I have kept up with a great deal of what I learned at the Hippocrates Health Institute. Their ways with foods and juices are the bedrock of this book. Most importantly, I have been growing wheatgrass for juice, and growing sprouts and tray greens. For wellbeing, as well as eating raw and living food meals, I drink shots of wheat grass and at least a litre/nearly two pints of green vegetable juice every day! The benefits are so obvious that I keep up those habits and it is all far less daunting than it first seemed.

What I never do is feel guilty or punish myself when making silly choices. State of mind is as important as food for wellbeing. Do not season your food with guilt or any other negativity! Many people find they need to work on their states of mind and attitudes when they change to this way of eating. That kind of support is part of my work, whether it is about weight or other issues. As you upgrade your level of wellness through eating this way, you are likely to have more energy for doing the inner work. As you detox your body, you may have to detox emotional issues at the same time.

One personal story I can share about emotional and physical detoxing is from when I was first at the Hippocrates Health Institute. I joined a group session with a focus on emotional issues and put myself forward. In that one session I was able to break through to a much healthier way of seeing some difficult past events. In the break I went out and looked up at the palm trees. I realised that I was seeing much more clearly, *physically*. That clearer eyesight has stayed with me, and my eyesight stopped deteriorating.

Since then I have made many other emotional breakthroughs, and weathered changes that might have been much harder without this food. I hope eating this way supports you too.

What I am *not* is a raw chef. My experience is from making food at home, and teaching people how to prepare food to eat at home. I took these photos at home and the pencil drawings were done at the dining table by a friend. My daughter did the pen sketches and cover art and took the cover photo.

I have been inspired to write the book by people who asked for the recipes, and because I wanted to spread the recipes further afield, sharing them with all who will enjoy them and who want wellness.

When people show complicated tricks they say 'Don't try this at home.' Instead, I can wholeheartedly say exactly the opposite!

*Please do **try this at home!***

Good Ways To Start

- ❧ Buy plenty of organic salad vegetables
- ❧ Buy lots of lovely ripe lemons and use them for drinks and dressings
- ❧ Have at least one big mixed salad a day and make the dressing with lemon juice
- ❧ Buy packets of sprouts and eat plenty in every main meal
- ❧ Buy some seeds to sprout and make a start – lentils are really easy
- ❧ Treat yourself to a sharp knife and a good juicer – see the **Good Equipment** section
- ❧ Scout around the nearest independent health food shop for good ingredients, perhaps starting with tamari and nut butter
- ❧ Relish thoughts of how this wonderful food will enhance your life
- ❧ Focus first just on the recipes and information that most attract you, and come to the rest when you find your bearings and are ready for more

♧ Make at least one of these recipes today, and keep making more to expand your repertoire

Balance

People talk about 'balance', a 'balanced diet', and a balance between eating what is healthy *and* eating and drinking what you enjoy.

I hope this book will help update your idea of a balanced diet. I was brought up thinking a balanced diet meant eating meals with a portion of animal food for protein, potatoes/rice/bread for carbohydrates, and vegetables for vitamins and minerals.

This misleading view is rife in western cultures. You can more easily find a healthy nutritional balance in organic raw and living vegan foods than by eating meat and dairy foods that are harder to digest. There are proteins, vitamins, carbohydrates and minerals in different proportions in all plant foods.

Read on to learn about tried and tested ways of eating that can provide balanced nutrition, giving you much more energy and a greater sense of wellbeing.

The other way people often think of balance is in terms of the balance between *healthy food choices* on one hand and *choices for pleasure* on the other. I hope these recipes help you to re-think that one! Raw and living food from plants can be delicious, delightful, and downright healthy at the same time, the choice for pleasure as well as health.

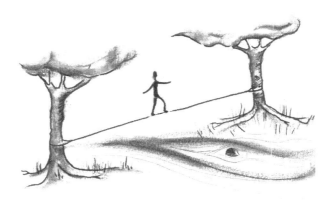

That is why you see the picture of a tightrope walker here. The healthier she is the more centered she can be, and the easier it is for her to balance. Read on to find out what does contribute to balance in life.

Vegetarians and Vegans

Vegetarian food is food without meat. Vegetarians often eat eggs, cheese, milk and butter, as well as vegetables, fruit and other plant foods. Some eat fish. To my mind eating fish is not being vegetarian, because fish are animals.

Some non-vegetarians assume vegetarians eat fish, which on occasion gives non-fish-eating vegetarians some explaining to do!

Vegan is a shortened form of the word vegetarian, and it describes food and people who eat food wholly from plants. Vegan food has been marginalised, put down over the years and judged as lacking. This is partly because it has been drummed into us that we need animal protein because it is 'complete'. People have seen vegan foods as lacking complete protein. Attitudes to vegan food are changing however, as vegetarian food becomes more popular. These days it shows up on most restaurant menus. The guidelines in this book are around vegan food.

Protein refers to a group of amino acids, the most important of which are called the essential amino acids. A steak has them all and a hazelnut has most of them. However, the essential amino acids do not all have to come from the same item of food and they do not all need to be present in each meal, as long as they are all included in each 24 hours. A well-balanced vegan diet has all the essential amino acids.

More health problems are in fact caused by eating too much protein, particularly animal protein foods, than by eating vegan food. Of all age groups, babies need the most protein. Later we are no longer growing at that rate and simply do not need as much.

Vegan food is cheaper to produce than vegetarian food and meat. Less waste and pollution is created and much less land is required than for grazing animals. If a burger ends up cheaper than the salad in the bun, it is because of government subsidy. Animals raised for food have huge carbon hoof prints! They present the world with a bigger problem than air travel.

For the sake of our environment, should we all be serious about eating more food from plants? Because food from plants costs so much less and uses fewer natural resources, we do not need to create Frankenfoods, such as genetically-modified food and artificial meat, in order to feed the human race. If you want to live lightly on the planet consider this way of eating.

Well-prepared vegan food really is easier to digest than food from animals. This may be hard to swallow if your experience of vegan food has been of heavy cooked nut roasts and bean dishes, but it is true!

Good Organic Food

There are two main reasons why organic food is better for you.

1. Organically-grown plants are not sprayed with potentially toxic pesticides and other chemicals. This minimises the toxic load on your body, so you can get on with healing and living life to the full. On the whole, being well is cheaper than getting ill.
2. Better care is taken of the soil so that it provides a richer array of nutrients in a natural balance for the plants, and hence for you.

Comparisons between organically and conventionally-farmed foods often show better levels of nutrients for organics. Organic produce might cost more, but is likely to provide more nutrition.

The peels and skins are usually highly nutritious, but polluting chemicals tend to be concentrated in surfaces, such as in apple peel and carrot skin. It is scary that British government guidelines recommend peeling carrots! Even the dirtiest organic carrot only needs a quick scrub before grating or slicing, and, since you are lovingly preparing your food, why would you peel off a nutritious layer? Avoiding the expense of buying organics might be a false economy if you have to throw away more of the conventionally-farmed produce and it provides less nutrition.

Buy as much organic food as you possibly can. What if that is a stretch for your budget? With some items it is even more important than others.

Among plants, the herbs are so full of essential oils that insect pests are less interested in them. They get sprayed less than regular vegetables such as lettuces, or not at all, so you are probably OK with fresh herbs that are not organic. If you cannot grow your own, at least you will have the nourishment and taste of herbs.

The Environmental Workshop Group in America, see **Good Resources,** came up with a *Dirty Dozen* fruit and vegetables that receive the most chemical sprays – some with over 60 chemicals, and a *Clean 15* which receive the least spray.

If 100% organic is not possible for you yet, and you live in America, you could buy organics from the Dirty Dozen and your all-important produce for green juice, and cut corners for now by buying non-organic for the Clean Fifteen.

Dirty Dozen
Highest in pesticides, starting with the highest:

1.Apples	5.Spinach	9.Potatoes
2.Celery	6.Nectarines	10.Blueberries
3.Strawberries	7.Grapes	11.Lettuce
4.Peaches	8.Sweet red peppers	12.Kale/collard greens

Buy these organic

Clean 15
Lowest in Pesticide, starting with the lowest:

1.Onions	6.Peas	11.Cabbage
2.Sweet Corn	7.Mangoes	12.Watermelon
3.Pineapples	8.Aubergine	13.Sweet potatoes
4.Avocado	9.Cantaloupe melon	14.Grapefruit
5.Asparagus	10.Kiwi fruit	15.Mushrooms

Far better is to buy *all* organic, so you give your system as few new problems as possible.

Where – and When – Can I Get Good Food?

As far as possible, source fresh food that is in season, locally grown and organic. Eating cheaper produce in season brings costs down. So does your choice of dry goods. By looking around you may find organic food as cheap, or cheaper than, non-organic. Choose wisely: organic sunflower seeds are cheaper than organic macadamia nuts!

Depending on where you live, there are choices:

Grow your own
Make the best use of your garden, terrace, deck, window box or allotment. Create an organic indoor sprout farm on windowsills and shelving.

Pick wild food
Find plants away from roads and sprayed lands. To play safe, stick with plants you know, learn on an expert-lead foraging outing or get an identification book with photos. Start with young stinging nettles in green juice, or serve young dandelion leaves and flowers with the **Hippocrates House Dressing**. Wild food is often incredibly nutritious, in part because the soil has not been touched by agriculture.

Join a Community Supported Agriculture Scheme (CSA)
These are getting popular in the States, the UK, Europe and Australasia. People buy shares in the farm and get a weekly vegetable share in exchange. Some put in hours of work in exchange for their food. It is a very good way to get greens in season. Prices compare with supermarkets and the food is likely to be fresher and of better quality. Bursary schemes may be available and you may be able to negotiate to get a share of specific seasonal vegetables and herbs for your raw cuisine.

Make a regular organic vegetable box order
That way you can get a weekly box of vegetables delivered to your door. Some suppliers are local market gardeners. If so, ask them for some of the carrot, celery and beet tops that they usually compost. Put the tops

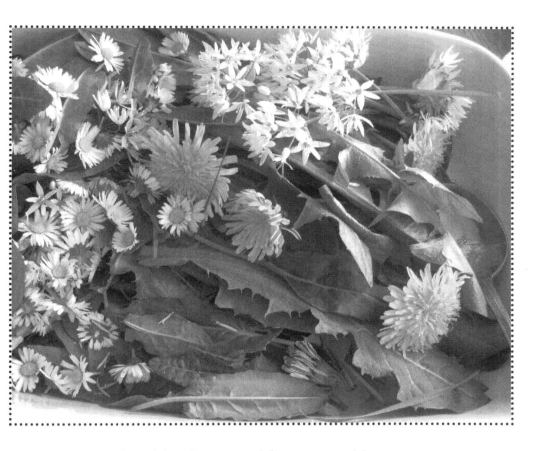

Dandelion leaves and flowers, sorrel leaves,
daisies and wild garlic flowers.

in your green juice and put the beetroot tops in juice or salad. Some suppliers may let you tailor your order to suit your juicing and raw food needs.

Go to farmers' markets
Hopefully you will find hardy grower-stallholders who picked their organic produce the afternoon before, and got up early for you. You should find interesting varieties of vegetable. Look for vegetables with their tops still on. Stallholders may be happy to give you discarded green tops from the back of their stall for your green juice. Many local farmers use few or no pesticides and so it is worth talking to them even though their banner does not say organic. It costs money to be Certified Organic.

Go to greengrocers
Ask for organics. That way you raise consciousness.

Go to good independent health food shops
These are increasing their ranges as awareness of raw food grows. They may have fresh organic food and good raw ingredients such as unpasteurised miso, unheated nut butters and raw dried seaweed. Check the small print to make sure things have not been heated. Do not expect everything they sell to be healthy. They cater for all tastes, dietary requirements and levels of wellness knowledge.

Go to the supermarket
They are not my top choice as the fresh food may not be that fresh, plus you get wasteful plastic packaging, but they sell some organics. Adapt a planned menu to suit their organic bargains.

Go online
There are plenty of companies ready and willing to sell you just about every specialty raw food on the planet. Work out what you need and what is worth paying for. Perhaps buy some dehydrated crackers in order to get ideas for your own, but unless you are money-rich and time-poor you

can buy the ingredients for creating your own delicacies more cheaply. The sweet raw treats may not be that helpful for wellness. Things I get online include dried seaweed, blue-green algae powder, chlorella, spirulina, raw rice protein powder, and grains and seeds for sprouting. Buying online in bulk and comparing between suppliers saves money. See **Good Resources.**

Good Ingredients

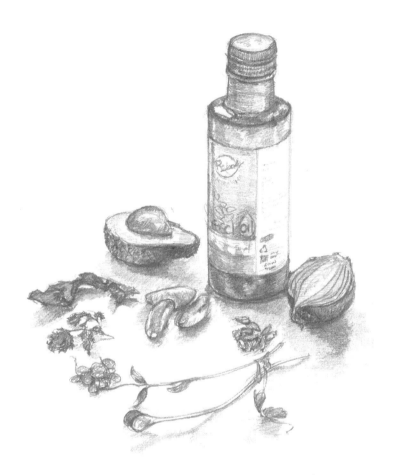

Avocado, hemp oil, onion, snow pea green, sunflower green,
Brazil nuts, wheat berries, lentil sprouts, coriander and
seaweed.

Blessings on the blossom
Blessings on the fruit
Blessings on the leaves and stems
And blessings on the root
Traditional children's grace

Have all these:
- Sprouted seeds and beans
- Tray-grown greens
- Vegetables
- Nuts and seeds, soaked and sprouted
- Grains, soaked and sprouted
- Wheatgrass juice
- Algae – spirulina, chlorella and AFA/blue green algae
- Fermented foods
- Oils and fats
- Fruit
- Herbs and spices, including herb teas

I use the British names in this book, Here are some US equivalents:
Courgettes = Zucchini
Aubergines = Eggplants
Coriander = Cilantro
Spring onions = Scallions
Snowpeas are the same as UK mangetout, except that for the pea shoots rather than the edible peapods, people call them snowpeas in the UK *and* in the US

Sprouted Seeds and Beans

Lentil sprouts, aduki sprouts, mung bean sprouts, Chinese bean sprouts, alfalfa sprouts, broccoli sprouts, mustard sprouts, cress sprouts, radish sprouts, fenugreek sprouts, sprouts, sprouts, sprouts. These life-filled baby plants are at the heart of the raw and living food way of eating. Happily more and more are on sale in health food shops and supermarkets now, so having a busy life is no excuse for not eating them in *every* main meal! They take about two and a half hours to digest.

Tray-grown Greens

Snow pea greens, sunflower greens and buckwheat lettuce. These grown-on sprouts are also at the heart of this way of eating. Grow plenty or get trays delivered to you. They take about two and a half hours to digest.

Vegetables

Avocado, Asparagus, Acorn squash, Arugula, Beetroot tops & roots, Broccoli, Bok Choy, Brussels sprouts, Butternut squash, Cabbage, Carrots, Cauliflower, Celery, Chard, Chinese cabbage, Courgettes, Cucumber, Corn salad, Celeriac, Collard, Dandelion, Daikon radish, Endive, Fennel, Green beans, Garlic, Interestingly shaped roots, Jicama, Kale, Kholrabi, Lambs' lettuce, Leeks, Lettuce, Mushrooms, Nettles, Onions, Parsnips, Peas, Purple sprouting broccoli, Quickly juiced greens, Radish, Red capsicums, Rocket, Scallions, Shallots, Spinach, Spring onions, Swede, Sweet corn, Sweet potato, Sweet red pointed peppers, Spring greens, Turnips, Uncooked all of these, Very fresh green leaves, Watercress, Yams, Xceptionally good fresh produce, Zucchini.

In the vegetable world you can write with a living alphabet.

All of these vegetables taste good prepared in raw ways, as do all the others available in different places around the world. I doubt there is one here that does not have particularly good nutritional and healing benefits. They all draw up precious minerals from the soil and hold treasure stores of enzymes, vitamins, protein, carbohydrates and water in an ideal form. They take about two and a half hours to digest.

Here are notes on just some:

All the green leaf vegetables are wonderful in salads and green juice, adding so much variety, texture and flavour. The green colour is the chlorophyll made in sunlight that is *essential* for wellbeing.

Avocados are a vegetable-like fruit, but they combine so well with vegetables that you can treat them like a vegetable – and like a fruit.

The cabbage family, and broccoli especially, have particularly good immune system support and anti-cancer properties. Watercress and broccoli deserve special mention as vegetables that have shown up well as healers in cancer studies. I suspect that, many, even all, of the other food vegetables would show up well too in a variety of ways, if they were made the subjects of clinical studies.

Carrots and beetroot add sweetness and are good in moderation – better used in dishes rather than juiced so you do not over do the sugar. Put the tops in juice. Slice fresh beetroot stalks and leaves finely for salads.

Courgettes have a mild taste that complements other foods well. Grate them as raw 'rice', blend them as a thickener and make them into thin strips for wonderful raw 'pasta'.

Cucumber is a favourite salad vegetable that can be cut in so many attractive ways, including making it into pasta strands. Put plenty in green juices.

Garlic and onions add fantastic savoury taste. That lovely cooking smell of onions and garlic is the smell of the essential oils leaving town. Use much less in raw food and the flavour will still be intense. I use milder varieties of onion such as the little red onions I can find easily in Britain, and very finely sliced leeks, spring onions and shallots.

Peas, finely sliced beans and asparagus add good tastes and crunch. If you marinate them, and perhaps soften them slightly in a dehydrator, they become more like stir-fried vegetables.

Parsnips, courgettes and celeriac can be grated as raw 'rice'.

Radishes and long white daikon radishes can be grated, sliced, and even made into raw 'noodles'.

Sweet corn is so delicious raw that I wonder why I ever cooked it! Sadly, much is now grown from genetically modified strains, particularly in the US. It is important to buy only organic corn and to check that it is definitely GMO free.

Sweet potatoes are a better nutritional choice than potatoes. You can make them into angel-hair 'pasta' for savoury dishes or steam them if you have some cooked food.

Two particularly healthful fungi are shitake and reishi mushrooms.

Ripe red capsicums, red bell peppers and red sweet pointed peppers are interchangeable in the recipes. They are *not* interchangeable with the green ones, which are unripe and make more work for your system. All peppers are in the same questionable family as potatoes, aubergines and tomatoes, and some choose to avoid them all. Red peppers are much less acidic than tomatoes and milder on the system. They are a good alternative to tomatoes, for example when blended with lemon juice in a raw pasta sauce.

Edible Flowers

are lovely for garnishing and decorating savoury and sweet dishes. Pick them from pesticide-free sources. Try these:
Nasturtiums, blue borage flowers, wild pansies and violets, marigold petals, common lawn daisies, rosemary flowers, red and white clover, elderflower petals, wild rose petals, dandelion flowers, sage flowers, thyme flowers, marjoram flowers, ramsons (wild garlic) flowers, chive flowers and carnation petals.

Many flowers are poisonous, so stick to those you *know* are safe.

Nuts and Seeds

Pumpkin seeds, sesame seeds, sunflower seeds, hemp seeds, flax/linseed seeds, chia seeds, Mila, poppy seeds…

Brazil nuts, pecans, almonds, walnuts, pine nuts, pili nuts (in the Philippines), macadamia nuts, hazelnuts, coconuts…

Nuts and seeds are concentrated: compared to sprouts and vegetables, we only need small amounts. They give meals substance and are rich in protein and helpful oils/fats. Seeds are generally from smaller plants, and nuts from trees. Eat a good variety, and make sure they are fresh and raw. If the sunflower or sesame seeds you buy will not sprout, they are not viable live seeds. Find a different source. Ask for raw nuts and seeds. Soak, and perhaps sprout them briefly, to vastly increase their nutrition and ease of digestion. They take about four hours to digest.

Coconuts are wonderful when young, green and fresh, but the older brown-shelled ones are less helpful and are frequently rancid. You can buy raw young coconut juice in cartons.

Chia seeds and Mila™ are tiny South American seeds with a mild nutty taste that are good for thickening and enriching dishes. They soothe the digestive tract and have an incredibly potent nutritional profile with high antioxidant levels, complete protein, vitamins, minerals, phytonutrients and Omega 3s. Mila is a proprietary microscopically-sliced mixture of specific strains of chia seeds. Some health practitioners around the raw movement are excited to find that for energy, mental clarity, athletic endurance and improved digestion people respond even better to Mila than to chia seeds. Many people report that Mila makes a noticeable difference to their energy levels and recovery rate from illness. Chia seeds are usually sold whole and add interesting texture to sweet and savoury dishes such as **Carob Birthday Cake** and **Oatcakes**. I use Mila and chia seeds, and you will find plenty of recipes here that include them. You can buy Mila from my site: http://www.lifemax.net/judybarber/

Peanuts often have toxicity associated with them and are best avoided altogether.

Ordinary cashew nuts from health food shops are steamed to remove the shells and may be rancid and toxic. Look online for hand-cracked raw cashew nuts and be prepared for the cost. Perhaps use the raw ones occasionally for extra-creamy luxury sauces and desserts, but stick with the other nuts for day-to-day nutrition.

Nut and Seed Butters

You can buy tahini (sesame seed butter) and butters made from ground almonds, Brazil nuts, hemp seeds, pumpkin seeds, walnuts, sunflower seeds and others. Check they are raw. They are convenient, have interesting textures and have many good uses. Making almond mayonnaise is very quick with almond butter. Bought butters are usually not soaked and dehydrated before grinding into butter, so making your own with the grinder parts on an auger juicer is a better option, see the **Nut Butter** recipe.

Oils and Fats

There is plenty of good oil/fat in soaked/sprouted nuts and seeds, and in avocados. You do not actually need additional fats and oils, but they can help with warmth and energy in a cold climate, and with keeping your weight up. They are delicious. Buy them organic and cold pressed. The best for nutrition are olive, walnut, pumpkin, hemp, flax/linseed and sesame oil (not toasted). Flax/linseed oil and hemp oil are particularly beneficial because they provide the essential omegas.

Oils/fats take about four hours to digest. The oils in these recipes are those that tasted right at the time, but do ring the changes amongst those best oils for nutrition. Sunflower oil and safflower oil are of less value because they do not have such superior nutrition.

Forget margarine. It is a factory food that is often made from rancid heat-treated oils that are blended, bleached, deodorised, whipped, oxidised and flavoured. Instead, try some of the raw butter and spread recipes in **Good Patés, Spreads and Side Dishes**

Opinions vary on raw coconut oil. It is a saturated fat and not part of the Hippocrates way. It is in a few of these recipes, but I use it less and less, and do not miss it. More recently I thicken sweet treats with chia seeds/Mila or psyllium husks instead.

Fermented Foods

If you give up dairy food it is goodbye to yoghurt with its millions of helpful bacteria, but you can eat millions of helpful bacteria in different naturally fermented plant forms.

The fermented soy foods are miso, tamari, nama shoyu, shoyu and tempeh.

Look for *unpasteurised* on the label so you know the bacteria are still alive! In fermentation the soybean is changed radically and becomes easy to digest, unlike factory-produced soya products such as soymilk. Miso, tamari, nama shoyu and shoyu are delicious condiments, but go gently to avoid having an unhealthy amount of salt.

Miso is a salty savoury paste with a complex interesting taste that is wonderful in sauces and soups. Sweet white and sweet brown miso are fermented for a shorter time and have lighter, sweeter, tastes than the darker brown aged misos. Look for *sweet* miso and *aged* miso in the recipes.

Tamari was traditionally the liquid from the top of the jars of fermenting miso and should be wheat-free. Nama shoyu and shoyu are fermented in a similar way, but from a mixture of soy beans and wheat.

Tempeh is a cake of fermented soybeans that is a good addition to savoury dishes when it is marinated and perhaps lightly dehydrated. See **Tempeh Pieces with Garlic.**

The two common fermented vegetable pickles are European pickled cabbage **Sauerkraut** and spicy Korean **Kim Chi**. Make your own or buy them from the chiller in a good health food shop, checking they are unpasteurised, and hence live.

Grains and Grain-like Seeds

Grains such as wheat, rye, barley, sweet corn, rice and oats are grass seeds from grasses with long thin leaves. All are starchy, providing plenty of slow-release carbohydrates for sustained energy. This is very different from the instant energy hits of sugary plants such as dates or sugar cane, which can send blood sugar levels all over the place.

Some grains, wheat especially, are somewhat acidic and contain gummy gluten that can be hard to digest. It was the original chewing gum and it may literally stick around in the gut causing problems. When you sprout wheat the biochemistry changes and it becomes easier to digest. There is no gluten in wheatgrass juice because it is made from the grass and not the grain.

You can buy or make sprouted Essene bread as a good bread alternative. Oats have less gluten than wheat but it is hard to find them raw. Most oat groats and rolled oats have been steamed. Hunt for raw ones. See **Good Resources**.

Brown rice is at best neutral. I serve it cooked sometimes. There is not much food value in white rice or white flour. Why would anyone bother to eat either of these, once they know that?

Grain-like seeds include buckwheat, quinoa and millet. Grain-like seeds are fine foods providing plenty of complex carbohydrates. They have no gluten. They grow on plants with branching stems and wider leaves. They have more protein than grains, but are very starchy and best eaten at different meals from nuts and seeds. The beauty of millet, quinoa and buckwheat is that they are alkalinising and are very good alternatives to the ubiquitous wheat products -bread, pasta, cake and pastry.

Quinoa and buckwheat sprout easily and I personally like them better than sprouted grains. When they have just started sprouting they are interesting salad ingredients. Try them in nori rolls instead of rice.

I have failed to sprout millet in the UK, but I soak it overnight to start its growth process, before cooking it as I would a grain.

Grains and grain-like seeds take about two and a half hours to digest.

Sea Vegetables/Seaweeds

These are crucial raw foods. Seaweed and sea vegetables are exactly the same plants, with different names. They grow on rocks near the surface of oceans where they receive sunlight. They are strong flexible plants that can withstand tides. Imagine that strength and flexibility in your body. Buy them dried or fresh packed in sea salt, or find them fresh in the wild.

The golden rules for harvesting seaweeds are:

* ❧ Pick from unpolluted places
* ❧ Do not over-pick in a potentially destructive way
* ❧ Only harvest what appears fresh
* ❧ Avoid purple seaweed unless you know what kind it is. A few of the purplish ones are poisonous, so do your homework. All the brown, green, and white varieties are edible

Some good ones are sea salad mixtures, nori, dulse, New Zealand karengo and kelp. Nori often refers to thin pressed sheets of nori for wrapping around savoury ingredients for Japanese-style nori rolls. These are a wonderful raw food. Oddly, nori is dark purple, but goes green when toasted. Most nori sheets are sold toasted but you can find untoasted sheets. Kelp is thicker, rubbery seaweed. It is good to have that as well as dulse and other lighter types, but I prefer it ground as a condiment. See the **Seaweed Sprinkles** recipe. You can also buy various ready-ground seaweed condiments.

Have seaweed with every main meal, sprinkled on, soft as a side dish, crunchy from the dehydrator or mixed into salads and dehydrated foods.

Spirulina, Chlorella and Blue-green Algae

The nutrition in these superfoods is quite incredible and they are important pieces in the raw and living food jigsaw puzzle. Use them for alertness, steady energy and stamina and appreciate their high protein, vitamin and mineral content. Add them to drinks and smoothies and try the **Green Crisps** recipe.

Herbs, Spices and Condiments

These wonderful ingredients transform the tastes of dishes in an infinite variety of ways and can be important for nutrition. Some overlap into herbal medicine, in a very safe way if used in normal amounts. Read up on their potentially healing qualities. For example, turmeric is hailed in studies as an anti-inflammatory medicinal spice to rival conventional medicines, and cinnamon and oregano are said to support the immune system.

A herb is usually a green leaf and a spice a stem, root or seed, often dried and ground to powder. You will find most of the herbs and spices below in these recipes. Try all of them.

Common, and not so common, culinary herbs include basil, coriander, parsley, mint, chives, dill, oregano, sage, thyme, rosemary, marjoram, tarragon, horseradish, borage and fennel.

Spices include ginger, turmeric, cayenne pepper, chili, cinnamon, cardamom, cumin, caraway, star anise, celery seed, coriander seed, cloves, lemongrass, mace, nutmeg, wasabi, mustard, and sumac.

Black pepper can irritate the intestinal lining. Instead use pinches of dried ginger, cayenne pepper and garlic powder to point up flavours. In tiny quantities they do that without being distinctive or hot.

Psyllium husks do not taste of much, but I was not sure where else to put them! These processed seed husks work brilliantly as thickeners in raw dishes. They are not raw, but so little is used and they are so mild that it does not matter. They are sold in health food shops and Indian delicatessens as a gelling agent for intestinal health and regularity, and are cheaper in the Indian shops.

Salty Tastes

We need salt, sodium chloride, for our inner ocean, but not much. Avoid processed table salt because it may have chemicals added so that it pours easily, and it will not have a range of minerals along with the sodium chloride. Celtic, and any salt from the sea, contains a range of mineral salts that provide a better balance than table salt, but still with a lot of sodium chloride. Himalayan salt is sea salt from ancient times.

Olives are pickled in salt and so are umeboshi plums, the vegetables for **Sauerkraut** and **Kim Chi** (see recipes), and the soya beans for miso, tamari and nama shoyu. Braggs Liquid Aminos sauce and Marigold Liquid Aminos sauce are salty. Those two are good savoury alternatives to the fermented Japanese sauces, tamari, shoyu and nama shoyu. Sea vegetables contain salt. Processed foods are usually too salty, and too much salt is a health hazard! Too little would be a hazard, but that is unlikely when there is even salt in a stick of celery.

Opinions vary as to how much salt is too much. In the raw food world some favour sea salt, including Himalayan salt, and some favour salt in fermented soy sauce – tamari and nama shoyu.

At the Hippocrates Health Institute the salty tastes offered are in seaweed/sea vegetables, in olives, in tamari/nama shoyu and in unfermented liquid aminos. I follow that lead, but use a little sea salt sometimes for a change. However, in the long term it is better to mainly enjoy the salty taste of the sea vegetables, and of the land vegetables.

Himalayan salt comes in pink and black. The black, in fact a cloudy pink colour, has a sulphur taste. A very tiny pinch can be good in dishes similar to traditional egg dishes.

The taste of tamari, nama shoyu and liquid aminos goes a long way. You seem to get more taste for the actual amount of salt in the sauce. I use tamari in the recipes because it is wheat free, fermented and because I enjoy the taste, but you can ring the changes.

Go gently. Let the flavour of the food speak for itself. When I write 'season to taste', that is not encouragement for a lot of salty seasoning. Some of the suggested quantities in my recipes are from earlier in my raw journey. My tastes are changing and I use less now. Gradually reduce the saltiness of your food, and make some savoury dishes without any sea salt or tamari/nama shoyu/liquid aminos. See the **Celery Salt** recipe for some raw plant saltiness to use instead of sea salt and tamari.

Good Superfoods

Superfoods are food ingredients and are just as helpful as they have always been. Many have been revered as food and medicine in traditional cultures, and now research is confirming their especially helpful properties. Which foods get classified as superfoods is likely to be a function of how much research has been done on each one as much as of how beneficial it is.

Here are some of my current favourites:

Blackcurrants, watercress, turmeric, blueberries, pollen, sage, thyme, oregano, Mila/chia seeds, blue-green algae, spirulina, chlorella, maca and avocados.

People who get into superfoods find a whole galaxy of powders, dried foods, tinctures and dried leaves. It is an expanding galaxy, and the hunt continues for another and another superfood. Some are brilliant.

I notice two commonly held beliefs about them:

* You need lots in order to be healthy
* There is a specific one that will make all the difference

Try some if you wish, but be wary of neglecting the super benefits of everyday raw and living meals with humble vegetables, sprouts, nuts and seeds for a cupboard of expensive rare imported powders. Until recently no one had the run of all the ideal foods on the planet, and we still do not need them all.

Supplements

You probably need some, especially vitamin B12. This is because we have so much to deal with in modern environments, and even organic soils can lack what we need.

A supplement such as an effervescent vitamin B and C tablet dissolved in a glass of filtered water might be an OK emergency measure, but only because it is stimulating the system, not because it is nourishing you.

The important distinction to make is between supplements made from *whole foods* and supplements made in *chemical processes*.

The former can make a positive difference. The latter frequently do not, and may create further imbalances because they are single chemicals that do not provide the synergy of natural plant ingredients. A common example is of chemically-produced ascorbic acid, which is only one part of the vitamin C that can be sourced from rose hips, acerola cherries, and in raw and living foods.

See **Good Resources** for a book on the subject by Dr Brian Clement.

Fruit

The problem with fruit is that it is full of sugar, which not only challenges blood sugar levels but tends to create acidity in the body. Older domestic varieties of fruit were less sweet than modern hybrids, so the vast quantities of fruit juices and sweet fruit consumed today are not really natural. Can you let fruit be an occasional treat? Try it as a breakfast sometimes, as a snack on its own or as a dessert much later than the main meal.

*Plea*se get the ripest fruit you possibly can. If you eat fruit that is not ripe, your system has to supply what is missing to balance it out. That can deplete you. Ripening fruit on sunny windowsills helps, but is not ideal.

Lemons and limes are wonder fruit that taste deliciously acidic but are alkalinising. They are fantastic in dressings, sauces, desserts, and in any dish that needs a twang. They are fine in both protein rich and carbohydrate rich savoury meals.

Avocados are fruits, just not sweet ones. They combine with any fruit and vegetables and are an incredibly healthy food. They are quite rich so perhaps have them about three times a week rather than every day.

Oranges are not alkalising in the body, unlike lemons and limes. I use orange juice and peel in sweet dishes occasionally for flavour, but know they are not the best foods for wellbeing. For an orange taste in a salad, try adding very finely-grated orange zest and lemon juice.

Tomatoes are fruit, strictly speaking, and not vegetables. At Hippocrates they serve them as a fruit treat for people who are avoiding sugar. I know cancer survivors who completely avoid tomatoes. I occasionally enjoy tomatoes when they are vine-ripened and are in dishes I am given when out. They are not in this book because they are so acidic. Instead there are salsa and sauce recipes using sweet red peppers and lemon juice.

Sweet red peppers are technically fruit, but are mild, and fine with vegetables. They take two and a half hours to digest.

Sweet fruits include all dried fruits and bananas, fresh dates and persimmons. Dried fruits are incredibly sweet: soak them first to dilute the sugar a little. Use rarely. They take about four hours to digest and are best eaten on their own, well away from other meals, and not that often! You will find raisins, sultanas and currants in my traditional Christmas treat recipes. Otherwise I rarely eat them.

Sub-acidic fruits include all the berries, peaches, cherries, pears, apples, nectarines, plums, lychees and papaya. They take a couple of hours to digest.

Acid fruits include pineapples, strawberries, pomegranates, kiwi fruit, cranberries, oranges, grapefruit and any sour fruit. They take about an hour to digest.

Melons digest so quickly that they are best eaten on their own. Mix different varieties together for melon salads, rather than mixing them with different fruit.

Sweet Ingredients

So many of us love sweet tastes and associate them with comfort, gifts and rewards. They are often viewed as treats, but are they really? Short term they are, and they may get us through emotionally tough times and exhausted moments. But can they really be treats if they do not help us to be full of life? How many people are sugar addicts, addicted to sugar in drinks, cakes, sweets, jams and pastries? Sugar is in cane sugar, beet sugar, corn syrup, fruit, agave syrup, maple syrup, honey and more. It is even in carrots and beetroots (so it is better to use them in meals rather than drinking a lot at once in juices). Even small quantities of sugar can upset blood sugar levels, so that an initial burst of energy is followed by a drop in energy or tiredness. Some research shows sugar implicated in candida and other health problems, and that it 'feeds' cancer cells. Sugar contributes to acidic body conditions, too acidic for a healthy metabolism. Read more in Dr Brian Clement's chapter in *Raw Food Works*, see **Good Resources**.

Alcohol creates the same problems as a sugar in the body, even with less-sweet drinks such as beer. Apparently, recovering alcoholics at AA meetings tend to go for the biscuits and cookies, another addiction.

Pure Stevia Extract is a safe herbal sweetener that actually helps to stabilise blood sugar levels! It contains no sugar and is top of my sweetening list. Use it as a powdered green leaf (if you like a leaf taste along with the sweetness, which I do not) or as a very concentrated liquid or white powder pure extract. Far less than a salt spoon is enough to sweeten a drink. It can be used in sweet and savoury dishes. Some find it goes better with some flavours with than others. See what works for you.

If you want to stay right off sugar for general wellbeing, or for weight loss or healing from candida, cancer or diabetes, stevia is a godsend. Make sure that you buy pure stevia extract rather than the common brands that include other processed ingredients that may not be helpful even if they are called natural. It is sold as a powder in a pot with a tiny spoon or in a dropper bottle. When I write 'tiny spoon' in the recipes I am referring to the tiny spoon in the stevia pot that you buy. In my nearest supermarket there is no pure stevia, but only pure stevia extract mixed with other highly processed ingredients. Some brands include other sweeteners and even sugar! See **Good Resources** for stevia online.

Yacon is a South American root, powdered or as syrup, that you can find on raw food websites. It is not cheap, but it is beneficial to helpful gut bacteria. Much of the sugar passes through the system unchanged. It is not such a bad choice in occasional sweet treats.

Carob powder is the sweet ground seedpods of a Mediterranean tree. Most in the shops has been roasted but you can find it raw online. It has a sweet caramel taste similar to chocolate. As a beneficial food with no caffeine, it is a good substitute for chocolate/raw cacao. Carob is such a good dessert ingredient that you can enjoy it in sweet treats, without missing the chocolate.

Agave syrup from a cactus is incredibly popular in raw recipes, but apparently it is always cooked during processing! Many now question its use. It is hardly better than ordinary sugar on the glycaemic index that measures how fast a sugar hits your blood sugar levels.

Xylitol is a popular processed sweet white sugary powder, extracted from birch trees. Chemically, it is a sugar alcohol, not sugar. It has about two thirds of the calories of table sugar and is relatively low on the glycaemic index. It is less destructive to tooth enamel than sugar, but it is highly processed and is a laxative. If a lot can stress the intestines that much, why might not little amounts stress them over time?

Maple syrup is maple tree sap reduced to syrup by boiling – so not raw. It is relatively low on the glycaemic index. I use it occasionally for the taste, but more often use natural maple flavour essence from the States. The flavouring is fantastic in sugar free **Hippocrates Nut Icecream**.

Dates are so full of fruit sugar that I suggest you avoid them except for rare treats. Try the fresh varieties, such as Medjool, because at least they are delicious and hopefully raw.

Honey and pollen are collected by bees, so some strict vegans avoid them. You can find pollen collected by human hands. I choose to use bee-collected pollen and honey, partly because bees are in trouble worldwide with veroa disease and insecticides. Bee pollination is essential for human survival. Beekeepers who treat bees well, and do not feed them refined sugar, need support.

Honey has more flavour, and is sweeter than agave. Instead of expensive heated agave syrup, consider using cold pressed organic honey. It is not brilliant because it is flower nectar *sugar*, but it does have benefits. If cold pressed, therefore raw, it retains qualities that support the immune and nervous systems. Honey is useful for occasional sweet dishes for special occasions. I occasionally use tiny amounts in savoury dishes and dressings to bring out other flavours. That touch of sweetness satisfies my sweet tooth.

Pollen is a superfood that is the reproductive substance of flowers, full of whatever is needed for new plant life. Apparently, it is life-sustaining and you could live on it indefinitely. I would not want to try that, but most days I have a spoonful of pollen grains all lovingly collected on the furry legs of foraging bees. Nibble it thoughtfully as a helpful treat straight from the spoon, mix it into nut milks or sprinkle it onto breakfast cereal.

Sweetening in the recipes

If you get on with pure stevia extract and want to minimise your sugar intake, you can use it in almost all these recipes. Often I put a sequence of yacon/stevia/honey/maple syrup/agave from which you can choose.

Fish and Fish Oil

Ocean fish concentrate what they take in from the water into their bodies. These days that includes mercury and other pollutants.

Farmed fish are often fed pellets made from ocean fish and abattoir waste. I read that it takes five ocean fish to feed a farm fish of the same size. If you choose farmed fish for environmental reasons, you probably did not want to know that.

Fish oils have been pushed commercially as sources of the omega oils we never used to know we needed. The oil is a fishing industry waste product and has to be treated to disguise the rancid taste. Millions of oil capsules are swallowed to increase brainpower. However, the mercury concentrated in the oil is extremely damaging – to the *brain*! The liquid peroxide used in processing has been shown to cause cancer.

Chia seeds/Mila and plant seeds and oils such as hemp and flax/linseed, give you plenty of the important omegas, minus the poisonous mercury. Use those in your raw meals, along with other brain-boosting plant foods.

Good Sprouts – The Living Main Dish

At the heart of this way of eating are *living* vegan foods. The magic of nuts, beans and seeds is that they can stay dormant for years, retaining the power to spring into life. Seeds from ancient Egyptian tombs have been sprouted.

Sprouting needs water and warmth. Then a remarkable transformation takes place. The life in the seed moves out to form a root system and a stem, leaves, flowers, fruit and more seeds. As the seed starts to sprout, the potential for patterning a complete new plant is awakened. A great deal of generalised material for growth is present in easily-assimilated forms. This means that edible sprouted seeds are highly nutritious and loaded with life enzymes.

Some nuts and seeds, such as almonds, just need soaking. With others you take things further by sprouting them. For a select exceptionally nutritious few, you go further again until they are a few inches high and turning into green plants. Then they are full of what the plant needs for further growth to maturity, including the all-important chlorophyll that is so much like our own blood. There are much higher concentrations of easily-digested nutrients at this stage than in mature plants.

Knowing this makes it possible to create a complete and healthy way of eating out of organic raw vegan food. People are encouraged to take plenty of the sprouts on offer at the Hippocrates Health Institute buffet as the main dish, and to add all the other vegetables and created vegan delicacies as side dishes. Life becomes much, much easier with living foods. This is why *living* foods are the main dish.

Soaking

Soak nuts and seeds such as almonds, hazelnuts, Brazil nuts, macadamia nuts, pecans, walnuts, sesame seeds, pumpkin seeds and sunflower seeds (bought with their hulls removed). Soak them for a day or over night and rinse well. Soak any seed, nut or grain before use, whether or not you sprout them. The longer you soak nuts the sweeter they become, and you can store them in filtered water in the fridge for several days.

Sprouting

A simple and cheap way to sprout seeds is in large glass jars with nylon netting and rubber band lids. Cut net circles bigger than the tops of the glass jars and hold them in place with the rubber bands. Or buy special glass sprouting jars with firm plastic mesh in their lids. Some lids have a helpful sidepiece so you can set them to drain at an angle. You can buy slightly larger plastic beakers with slits in the bottom that sit inside plastic beakers. These are good for travelling. Plastic stacking trays are good too. I suggest starting with glass jars and netting until you get used to things and know what you want. You can also buy electrical self-watering setups.

Easy seeds to start with are whole red lentils, green lentils, mung beans, alfalfa, clover and fenugreek. Then you can graduate to fussier seeds such as aduki beans, broccoli and black mustard. After soaking, rinse and drain the seeds twice a day until they start forming little roots, and (depending on the type) little shoots and their first seed leaves. Keep an eye on them on your counter top and keep them out of direct sunlight. Buy bags of sprouts as well so you can learn by comparing them with yours. Yours may be better!

Your mung beans will not grow to Chinese bean sprout size, although it is the same plant, because the long fat ones are grown weighted down in controlled conditions. Yours will put up with life on your kitchen counter and you will get crunchy little roots. I grow mine, and also buy the Chinese ones for variety.

Growing Tray Greens and Wheatgrass

This might seem complicated, but it becomes very simple. Any gardening experience you have will help you. The routine is an active meditation.

❧ For each two standard-sized plastic garden seed trays, the kind with draining holes, have one slightly larger tray for the tray of earth to sit in. Then you can contain the mess if you grow them indoors. The second seed tray is to use as a lid.

35

- Per tray, use approximately 2½ cups of grain/seed per tray for wheatgrass from spelt , ½ cup for sunflowers, ¾ cup for snow peas and ½ cup for buckwheat lettuce.
- Use topsoil or compost from your garden, or buy good quality compost or topsoil from a garden centre, preferably organic.
- Fill the trays with soil about an inch/2 centimetres thick.

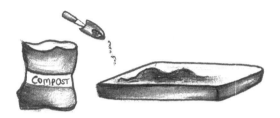

- Spread the sprouted seeds over the top.

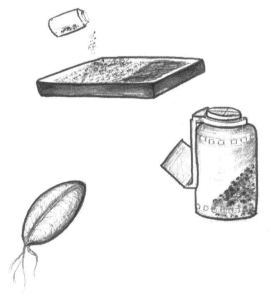

- Water very well and spray them with water.
- Invert another seed tray over the top as a lid to keep them in darkness.

❦ Let them grow for several days until the greens have grown tall enough to start pushing their lids up. This stage encourages them to grow upwards.

❦ Take the lids off. Then they can work with the light to create chlorophyll and continue to grow. Keep watering and spraying until they are ready to start harvesting at 5 inches/13 centimetres. Just harvest what you need and keep them growing for a few days.

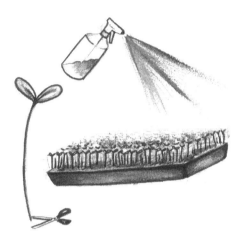

One good secret is that the plants are not fussy. If you are away, busy or forget to water them, they may still survive and flourish. You do not have to cut a whole crop at once because they will happily sit for days while you cut them handful by handful as you need them. Cut and keep in the fridge in plastic bags before the sunflowers start growing true leaves and the snow peas get straggly. It is fun watching these baby plants grow, and showing visitors. People appreciate bags to take home. When you learn how, you can help others by example. Get your seeds and grains from a good supplier and save money by buying in bulk.

The main tray greens to grow to eat are sunflowers in their black seed cases, and snow peas. Ideally grow enough to put plenty in your **Green Juice**. Pick the sunflower seeds before they start to grow their first true leaves. You can also grow buckwheat in its seed cases, for buckwheat lettuce for salads. As with the sunflower greens, just grow it until the first two seed leaves are fully developed.

Keep the snow peas growing after you have harvested the main crop, and you may get a second, smaller, crop.

You can grow wheat, spelt or barley grains for juicing wheatgrass. My preference is for spelt. It grows well and quickly, and tastes the sweetest, but experiment to discover what suits you and your growing conditions. Sprout the grains in the same way as the seeds for greens, until little roots start to form. Then get them planted in trays as soon as you can.

Expect crops in a week to 10 days. All depends on the time of year, the seed, growing temperature, humidity, and how often you remember to spray and water.

Pick the wheatgrass when the blades are dividing into two. Then crop them as near to the earth as you can (the white part of the stem is full of lecithin and good minerals). You will know you have kept it in the fridge too long if it starts to turn to hay.

The benefit of the wheatgrass is in the first growth. There is not much point in re-cutting the seed tray 'lawn' again when it has grown further, however nice and green it looks. At that point it is ready for composting.

You can have wooden shelving units to hold the trays. In summer and in a warmer climate you can grow your seeds outside. You can buy mini-greenhouses from garden centres. In the States you can get indoor bay systems for growing your crops without soil.

Once you have your system going, this is a simple and easy process that need not be too precise. It is a relatively inexpensive way to ensure you have optimum nutrition and delicious salad ingredients always on hand.

A sprout farm is very nice to have at home, a new dimension in houseplants! Do keep in mind that you can go online and order your tray greens and wheatgrass all ready to harvest. See **Good Resources**.

Good Equipment

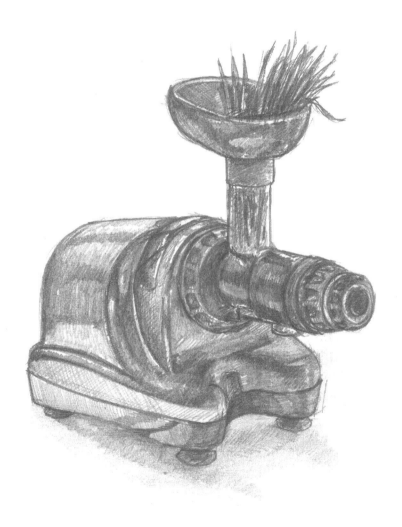

A single auger juicer

A Juicer

After a good knife, the most important equipment is a good juicer, one similar to the one in the drawing on the previous page. It is an auger juicer that crushes the juice out of the vegetables with one, or two, screw fittings in a narrow chamber.

By contrast, most juicers are centrifugal ones that grate the vegetables and spin them against a screen to separate the juice. As it spins round at high speed, the juice is oxidised more than in an auger juicer.

Green juice made this way is OK until you can get an auger juicer, but really you want the oxidation to happen when the juice is inside you! Then it can neutralise any free radicals on the loose in your system. Green vegetable juice (rather than fruit juice or fruit and vegetable juices mixed together) is ideal for alkalinising and detoxing.

This is juice without fibre that gives the digestive system a break from peristalsis (the muscular squeezing all through the gut) between meals.

You need a juicer that can tackle wheatgrass and green vegetables. On a very tight budget or when on the move, try a small metal or plastic single auger juicer such as the *Lexen Manual Healthy Juicer*, which is good for power cuts and holidays. Electric models I like are the single auger *Oscar Neo*, the *Omega* juicers and the *Angel*, a sturdy all-steel twin auger juicer. Compared to other juicers I have tried, there is less froth with the *Angel* and no fibre sludge in the juice. Apart from the Angel, twin auger juicers are more fussy to reassemble than single auger juicers, but do a better job and produce more juice. Have a look at the *Green Star* and *Green Power Kempo*.

These juicers crush out an incredible amount of juice and are very easy to clean and reassemble. This is important, because if you want the benefits of drinking wheatgrass and green juice you will be juicing every day, or perhaps several times a day.

A juicer is a big investment. Some choose the *Angel* because metal instead of plastic touches the juice, but it is more expensive and best just used for juice. A good thing about single auger juicers like the *Oscar/Omega* and some of the other twin augers is that they have other uses. You can make raw patés, ice cream and sorbet with them.

What you *must* do is get a juicer that copes with wheatgrass and green vegetables. Some juicers can only cope with fruit juice.

The benefits, in terms of wellbeing and energy, of drinking green juice and wheatgrass far outweigh the effort of juicing.

Knives

With sharp knives you can cut food more finely. They make a big difference to creativity and to how quickly you can work. Ceramic knives are expensive but good, and do not need sharpening. Some say food tastes better when cut with them and does not oxidise so quickly.

On the other hand, I bought two excellent knives in a bargain shop for a few dollars and they are a joy to use.

Learn how to use a knife sharpener to keep steel blades ultra sharp. You might find it helpful to have a small serrated knife as well.

A Blender

The *Vitamix* is at the top of the price range for rugged high-speed blenders for raw food enthusiasts. The *Blendtec* has a good reputation. These powerful blenders make velvet-smooth dressings, purees, soups and dips. The *Powermill* is good and much cheaper, but does not get things to quite the same velvet smoothness. Some of the highstreet brands are worth investigating and are far less expensive. Shop around as there always seem to be new brands coming on the market. Blenders are wonderful toys for preparing imaginative meals. Powerful high-speed blenders are no better for wellness than ordinary blenders because, although they blend things quickly, they whip in more air that oxidises the food. No blender avoids whipping air into the food, but they add so much interest and variety to raw food that I would not want to be without one.

On a budget, get your good juicer first, and use an ordinary blender for now. Read on to see whether you would rather spend first on a dehydrator, and wait for an expensive blender until you know enough to make the right choice for you. Try Ebay. I got a good *Vitamix* cheaply from a raw couple who had both brought a Vitamix to the relationship and now only needed one!

For making smaller quantities of very smooth creations, and to grind nuts, seeds and spices the *Tribest Personal Blender*, which comes with a grinding blade as well as a blending blade, is excellent. You get two small and two medium-sized goblets with screw lids for storing the dressing or whatever, or for taking your raw soup or smoothie to work. This may be all you need for one or two people.

A Food Processor

A food processor has many uses. Things usually have to be quite liquid to work in a blender but a food processor can handle thicker mixtures, and you can create a variety of interesting textures. *Magimix* is one good UK brand.

With a food processor you can make:
- Salsa and coarse dips
- Smooth spreads and patés
- Mixtures for flax crackers, corn chips, pizza bases and other dehydrated delights
- Sliced vegetables to dehydrate
- Dressings with an interesting grainy texture
- Vast quantities of chopped and grated salad ingredients
- **Almond and Date Marzipan**
- Nut or grain pastry for deserts, pies and quiches
- Thick smooth fruit desserts
- Cake mixtures

A Nut Milk Bag

This is a fine mesh bag with a drawstring, also called a jelly bag in cook shops. You can find them online. Use it for straining nut milks. You can also make wheatgrass or green juice with one (until you can have an auger juicer) by blending up the wheatgrass or vegetables in some water and straining them into a bowl. The wheatgrass juice you can strain straight into your glass.

A Dehydrator

I lived happily without a dehydrator for my first raw food year but now I would not want to be without one. Dehydrated food adds bite, crunch, interest and variety to your raw and living food life, and is wonderful indeed for making crackers, crisps and travelling rations, using up leftovers, drying fruit, making fruit leather for children, making alternatives to junk food, and for impressing guests! Dehydrated food retains far more enzymes than cooked food, even though it loses something by being oxidised over a long time.

A dehydrator is like a fan oven with more shelves, but one that can operate at much lower temperatures and with more air circulating. For raw food you operate it at about 115° F/46° Centigrade, which is as warm as possible without damaging the food, especially the enzymes. Lower than that and the food will take longer to dry out and the slim risk of bacterial contamination would be increased. This optimum temperature seals and dries out food quickly without damaging it.

Excalibur is considered to be the best brand. It has rectangular, not circular, trays. You can easily score mixtures into squares, rectangles or triangles. There is an even temperature, so everything dries out at the same rate and temperature.

Get the nine-tray, not the five-tray version, even if you are making food for one. You are unlikely to want to use it every day, and when you do use it you can make a lot and dry it all at once. That saves time and electricity. The other reason is that you may need to pull out some trays to give more depth for thicker things like patties, breads, kale crisps and burgers, and for drying seaweed and herbs.

With a built-in timer you can give something time to finish off while out or asleep. Humidity affects drying times. A timer lets you know how long certain things take to dry in your particular kitchen, so you can plan for next time.

In addition to the machine, you need non-stick drying sheets. These last for years. Buy them, at a price, with the machine, online, or buy rolls of silicone coated baking sheets from the supermarket and cut to size. These are for spreading out sloppy mixtures that would drip through the mesh. To save time, once the mixture has dried a little, you can turn the sheet over between two trays, peel it and then complete the drying straight on the mesh tray.

On a budget, you might want to get a dehydrator after a good juicer, and then save for a powerful blender.

Grinder

If your blender will not grind spices, nuts and seeds, you will need a coffee grinder or other small grinder. Or use the *Tribest Personal Blender* with the grinding blade.

Something for Making Vegetable Pasta

There are wonderful gadgets for making long thin strands of pasta from vegetables such as courgettes, sweet potatoes, carrots, daikon radishes and jicama. By turning a handle, vegetables can be transformed into long pasta threads. They are not cheap for hand-operated plastic gadgets, but they are great fun, and give you another way to be creative with raw food. The *Benriner* is versatile because it has fine, medium and coarse blades for different thicknesses and the *Saladacco* and *Spiralizer* are also good. I use my *Benriner* often to make courgetti dishes that are as soft and comforting as regular wheat pasta.

The cheaper way to make vegetable pasta is with a julienne cutter. This is like a potato peeler with small teeth and is quite quick to use. Skin it down the side of a courgette, skin and all, for long pasta strips.

Measuring Spoons and Cups

For raw food you do not have to be as precise as with some cooked dishes, except perhaps for cakes. Using measuring cups and measuring spoons is much quicker than weighing things and you can find them in cook shops. A regular tablespoon and teaspoon from your kitchen drawer and an old fashioned teacup are pretty much the same size as measuring spoons and cups. The standard sizes are:

5ml – teaspoon | 15ml – tablespoon | 250 ml – cup

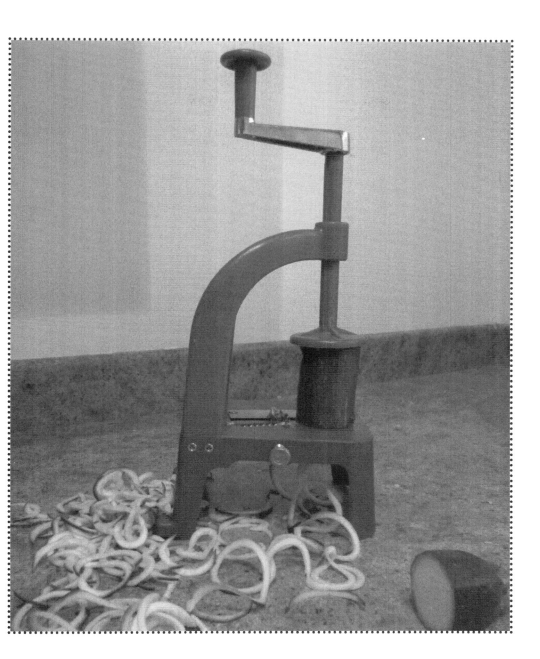

Making Raw Courgette Pasta with a Benriner

Good Food Combinations

When you follow food combining guidelines, food is digested easily and slips through the system in a healthy way. Fermentation can be avoided and the system is likely to be less sluggish.

Proteins and carbohydrates in raw vegan food are both important, but they need different mixtures of enzymes for digestion. It is not that proteins and carbohydrates together are *bad* for you, but eating them together makes more work for your system. That reduces available inner resources for getting on with life, or for dealing with health issues. This might not matter once in a while, but if you regularly eat meals that are *either* Protein rich or Carbohydrate rich you optimise the likelihood of reliable energy levels and wellbeing.

For example, if you go to a raw pot luck meal and try everything, regardless of food combining, you will probably get away with it and enjoy yourself tremendously, unless you are ill or run down. If you ate like that all the time you would still be better off than those who live on fast foods and ready meals, but you would be giving your system unnecessary hard work.

No meal can be completely devoid of protein or of carbohydrate. There is some of each in all this food. There are plenty of easily assimilable proteins and carbohydrates in sprouts and tray greens and I recommend you *always* include plenty in each meal along with raw vegetables, including sea vegetables.

The choice to be made for good food *combining* is between adding *protein rich* nuts or seeds, or *carbohydrate rich* grains or grain-like seeds. A tiny amount of one or other in a recipe, such as a little chia/Mila as a thickener, should not be a problem if you are well. Here are a couple of meals for examples:

A Protein rich meal:

A good selection of sprouts and tray greens. A mixed salad with lettuce, cucumber, radishes, and celery. **Almond Ranch Dressing**. Olives, soft dulse seaweed and **Kim Chi. Glazed Sunflower Twigs.**

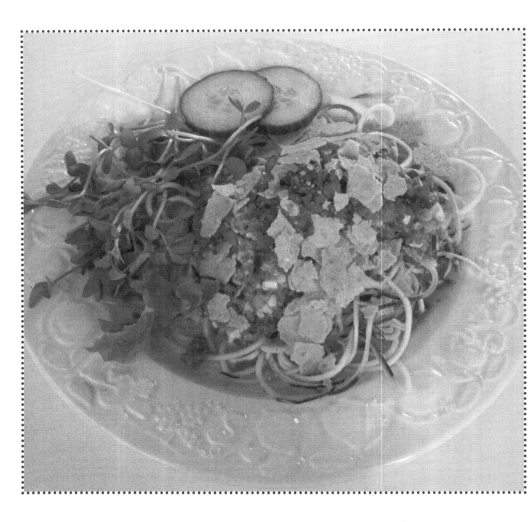

A protein rich meal of courgette pasta, Best Ever Pasta Sauce,
Sunflower Pecorino Shards, snow pea greens and
sunflower greens

A Carbohydrate rich meal:

A good selection of sprouts and tray greens with the **Hippocrates House Dressing**. **Sprouted Quinoa Tabouleh** with finely chopped parsley and sweet red pepper, garlic, lemon and red onion. Lettuce, olives, soft dulse seaweed and **Sauerkraut**.

Good Fruit Combining

For ease of digestion, eat fruit as a meal in itself rather than mixing it with vegetables. Preferably only combine like-with-like in one fruit group, sweet, semi-acidic or acidic, but you can combine them with the group next to them, so sweet and semi-sweet, or semi-sweet and acidic.

Avocado

As a fruit, avocado combines well with fruit for occasional treats. It combines equally well with vegetables, but it is so rich that you might want to have it at a savoury meal without much of either carbohydrate or protein. Two or three times a week is about right for avocados, not counting small amounts in sauces.

Now...

Turn to the start of the recipe chapters to find out how I have marked the recipes to make food combining easy.

Now you know about the ingredients, about the equipment and about which foods to combine, you can create your own brilliant banquets, buffets, dinner parties, family meals, picnics, romantic dinners, snacks, lunch boxes and perfect meals for energy, wellbeing and joy.

Bon Appetit! Enjoy your meal.

The
Recipes

Food-combining in the Recipes

To help you become familiar with food combining, I have written *Carbohydrate rich* or *Protein rich* next to some of these recipes. In one meal you can either have one or more carbohydrate rich dishes with any of the unmarked recipes; or have one or more protein rich dishes with any unmarked dishes. Or, you can have a meal with any of the unmarked dishes together. In those meals you might want to have some avocado.

It is interesting that so many of the dishes are Protein rich because they contain soaked nuts and seeds. You can see how easy it is to have enough protein with raw and living food! Remember that there is plenty of protein in sprouts and vegetables so you are unlikely to go short of protein.

I have not marked the **Good Sweet Treats** or **Muddled Good Sweet Treats** for food combining because they are intended to be eaten only occasionally and away from main meals. For good food combining, stick with the **Good Sweet Treats** rather than the **Muddled Good Sweet Treats.** Many of the sweet recipes can be made with pure stevia extract so that they do not create sugar problems in the body.

It is worth working with food combining to save your body some hard work and to leave more energy for the whole of your day. Try sticking to these food-combing guidelines for a while, and see what a difference it can make to wellness and energy levels.

Good Soups

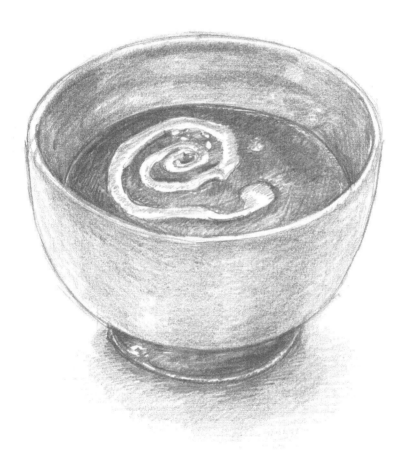

Warm Thai Red Pepper Soup with a swirl of
Sunflower Sour Cream

If your initial reaction is to imagine bowls of cold soup, think again. If the weather is cold and you want the comfort of warm food, warm but not cooked soups are perfect, and easy.

The basic equipment you will need is a knife, a chopping board and, for most recipes, a blender.

Any blender is fine, but for velvet smoothness the powerful high speed blenders are brilliant. The powerful ones can heat the soup by spinning it at high speed for rather a long noisy time. This is not ideal because in the process more air is whipped in, which further increases the antioxidant loss from the raw ingredients. Instead, blend the soup for as brief a time as possible to get the texture you want, and then warm the soup on a very low temperature on the stove, stirring with a clean finger – a reliable device for not overheating your soup!

The basic ingredients are vegetables, herbs, spices, seasonings, and perhaps sprouts, nuts and seeds. Avocado is a great addition for thickening soups and making them creamy.

Soups are a nourishing part of your raw recipe repertoire. They are far more satisfying nutritionally and to your taste buds than soups from a carton or tin. When someone is too unwell to chew or enduring dentistry they are a godsend. Soups are quick to make when hunger bites. They are easy to prepare ahead of time, but, for the least nutritional loss, are best blended at serving time.

These soup recipes will get you started, and then you can use whatever ingredients you have to hand to create an infinite variety.

Everyday Raw Soup

This is a very basic recipe from which you can create variations.

1 thick slice of onion	2 tablespoons unpasteurised sweet white or brown miso
1 clove of garlic	
2 medium carrots	A small piece of peeled fresh ginger
2 generous handfuls of green leaves such as spinach or lettuce	½ an avocado
½ a courgette	Optional: tamari to taste
2 cups filtered water	Sprigs of fresh herbs to taste

For 4 starter-sized servings:

Blend together everything except the avocado and the tamari. Taste, and add a very few drops of tamari to taste and the avocado, adding a little more water if you wish.

You could vary this by adding a few pitted olives instead of the miso, adding cold pressed olive oil and Italian herbs, or using a darker miso for a more hearty taste.

Warm gently and serve. Ta da!

Toppings for feeling tip top

To top things off you can swirl interesting herbs or creamy toppings on your soups, or serve them garnished with various sprinkles or croutons. Add tastes and textures, and add visual interest, with various toppings, garnishes and sprinkles. Here are some ideas to get you started.

- Finely chopped fresh herbs, such as chives, basil, coriander, tarragon and whatever else you have to hand
- Sprigs of freshly picked herbs
- Finely chopped salad leaves, in quantity, such as rocket, mizuna and watercress

- ✿ Crumbled dehydrated bread or cracker croutons
- ✿ Soaked sesame seeds or **Tastied Sesame Seeds** (see **Good Dehydrated Creations** chapter)
- ✿ A swirl of thinned dip or savoury nut/seed cream in a contrasting colour
- ✿ Drops of cold pressed olive oil
- ✿ **Browned Onions** or **Marinated Mushrooms**
- ✿ Finely sliced spring onions
- ✿ **Seaweed Sprinkles** or torn sheets of nori seaweed
- ✿ Blended herbs, spices and oil
- ✿ A grating of nutmeg
- ✿ A nasturtium flower or marigold petals

....

Carrot and Herb Soup

Carrot and coriander soup is an all-time favourite of mine, but carrot and basil, carrot and parsley, and carrot and mixed herbs are also good combinations. Serves 4

A large pinch of cayenne pepper
Optional: splashes of tamari
Up to 2 avocados
The juice of ½ a lemon
A Brazil nut-sized piece of fresh ginger
4 medium carrots
4 large handfuls of light herbs such as coriander, basil, and parsley
2 cups, + more as needed, of filtered water

Blend everything together with avocado, adding enough water to make it as thick as you like. Garnish with very finely chopped herbs, the variety you have used in the soup.

Pea Soup

This is a classic smooth soup, with the taste rounded out by the miso. It is a very good substantial soup for a cold day. Serves 4

2 cups of fresh or, if necessary, frozen peas, organic as always
3 cups filtered water
1 small clove of garlic
2-3 tablespoons unpasteurised aged miso
1 slice of mild onion
Optional: 1-2 teaspoons of cold pressed oil
A few sprigs of herbs such as basil, parsley and sage, or a sprig of mint

Blend all together till very smooth and adjust the seasonings to taste. Warm gently, stirring with your clean finger, to Goldilocks perfection. Serve in bowls warmed first with hot water.

....

Sea Chowder

Let this soup take you to a tropical island with coconut palms and fish swimming among the seaweeds in crystal clear water. Pick the seaweeds and make this soup. Serves 2

The juice and flesh of two young coconuts, or two cups of raw
  coconut water from a carton
A perfectly ripe but not squashy avocado
A handful of karengo or dulse seaweed
Optional: 2 teaspoons tamari
A generous squeeze of lemon or lime juice
½ – 1 cup of shitake mushrooms

A tiny piece of garlic
½ sweet pointed pepper or red capsicum, grated or very finely chopped
½ cup raw sweet corn scraped from the cob and lightly chopped
A small slice of mild onion

Tear the dulse or karengo in small strips and leave to soak in a little filtered water. Extract the juice and flesh from the young coconuts and blend it or the carton juice with the garlic, onion, lime or lemon juice.

Adjust the seasonings to taste, remembering that the seaweed will add saltiness. Add half the avocado and blend again to thicken the soup.

Chop the mushrooms and the rest of the avocado finely. Add them to the soup with the grated or chopped red pepper and sweet corn, and the seaweed, which should have soaked up all the water. If it hasn't, add the soak water too.

Leave for the flavours to mix, adding more liquid as necessary.

Serve at room temperature or gently warmed while stirring with a clean finger.

. . . .

Creamy Middle Eastern Soup
(Protein rich)

One day you might find a soup like this in an obscure raw roadside café on the road to Marrakesh. Serves 2

3 cups plain **Almond Milk,** preferably home made
2 ½ cups finely chopped mixed green vegetables such as broccoli, chard and asparagus
I thick slice of a small-medium mild onion
1 clove of garlic
1 teaspoon cumin seeds

A pinch of cayenne pepper
1 tablespoon unpasteurised aged miso
Optional: a splash of tamari
¼ cup of pitted kalamata olives
2 tablespoons cold pressed olive oil
1 tablespoon lemon juice
1 small bunch coriander leaves and/or 1 sweet red pepper, chopped
Filtered water

Blend all together, adding more water if too rich. Adjust the seasonings and serve at room temperature or warmed by stirring with a clean finger.

Olive Jar Soup

Olives, even raw ones, usually arrive soaked in salty brine, even when they are packed in olive oil. The salt is there as a preservative but it is a lot of salt to eat at once, especially if you like olives and want to eat quite a few! Fish out the olives and leave them in filtered water overnight, or until most of the sea salt has leached out into the water. Then put them back in cold pressed olive oil to keep in the fridge till they are used.

The water has a lovely olive taste that seems a pity to waste, so here is a recipe for the water! Serves 4

4 cups olive water (or, if that is too salty, a mixture of olive water and filtered water)	1 clove of garlic
	½ a small mild onion
	A pinch of cayenne pepper
2 medium carrots	1 tablespoon cold pressed olive oil
A handful of coriander and basil leaves	
	½ -1 avocado

Blend everything except the avocado. Add the tablespoon of oil. If it is too salty, add more water. Adjust the other ingredients and blend again.

Then add 1/2 an avocado or more to thicken.

This is a Mexican combination of flavours so it could be a starter for a Mexican meal, or you can turn it into a more substantial chowder by adding some of these:

- ♣ Raw sweet corn skinned off the cob and chopped a little to release the sweetness
- ♣ Finely chopped green vegetables and tray-grown greens, for example, lettuce and snow pea greens
- ♣ Finely chopped herbs such as basil, coriander and chives
- ♣ Finely chopped olives

....

Warm Thai Red Pepper Soup

I never had soup like this in Thailand, but the flavours are Thai favourites. Serves 4

Optional: A splash of tamari	1 large avocado
2 cups red capsicum juice (use the pulp to make a salsa or pizza topping)	½ an average cucumber
	½ a small red onion
	A small bunch of basil
2 cups filtered water	A small bunch Thai holy basil
2 tablespoons unpasteurised sweet miso	(if you can find it) and/or coriander
A pinch of cayenne pepper	A squeeze of lemon juice
2 cloves of garlic	Optional: a lemongrass stem or
A walnut-sized piece of peeled fresh ginger	a teabag or two of pure lemongrass.

Slice the lemongrass finely and make a tea with it by boiling the water and pouring it over the sliced lemongrass or teabags. Leave it to stew while you prepare everything else. Mix the capsicum juice in a saucepan with the miso. Crush or grate the garlic and ginger, and add them to the pan. Add the cayenne pepper. Chop the onion, cucumber and avocado as finely as possible and add them. Chop the basil and holy basil almost to a paste on a chopping board, and add them. Add a squeeze of lemon. Strain the lemongrass tea and add it to the pan. Stir all together and adjust seasonings and, if you wish, add a splash of tamari. Warm the mixture gently over a low heat, stirring with your clean finger until warm. Serve in bowls heated with hot water.

Asparagus Soup
(Protein rich)

I associate asparagus with smoothness, and find this soup a perfect way to appreciate the taste of asparagus in a smooth way. For a contrasting crunch, save the very tips of each asparagus shoot for a garnish. Serves 4

A small bunch of fresh
  asparagus
A small pinch of cayenne pepper
Optional: a pinch of sea salt or a
  splash of tamari
1 small clove of garlic
1 thick slice of mild onion
1 teaspoon dried thyme or 2 of
  fresh, chopped

A few sprigs of parsley
4 cups of quite dilute almond
  milk, home made if possible
2 heaped tablespoons hulled
  hemp seeds
6 sticks of celery
6 Brazil nuts

Break off the rough ends of the asparagus and save for green juice. Break off the tips of the asparagus and set aside. Blend the main parts of the asparagus shoots with everything else. Adjust the seasonings to taste.

Serve this soup cold, or gently warmed by stirring it with your clean finger over a low heat. It is delightful either way. Slice the asparagus tips very finely and sprinkle them on the soup at the last moment.

. . . .

Warming Miso-Vegetable Soup

You come in feeling cold and do not want a cold salad, but you do want a large bowl of warm, nourishing sustenance with complex flavours and something to chew on. This soup is a miso broth thickened with avocado and full of very finely chopped or minced vegetables. Use whatever vegetables you have to hand along with the garlic clove, small red onion and ginger. Serves 4 in large bowls

8 cups warm filtered water	4 level tablespoons
2 small cloves of garlic	unpasteurised aged miso
1 small mild onion, finely	6 cups (total) finely chopped
chopped	herbs, spinach, red capsicum,
2 avocados	celery, lettuce and other salad
2 walnut-sized chunks of peeled	greens
ginger	2 cups sprouted lentils

Crush the garlic, crush or mince the ginger finely and mix them with half the miso and a little water. Mash in half the avocado and stir in the rest of the water. Pour it all into a saucepan. For a stronger broth, pour a little of the liquid out, mix with more miso and return to the pan. Chop the other half of the avocado and everything else very finely and add to the pan. Warm gently, stirring with your clean finger. Serve in bowls warmed with hot water.

Good
Salad Dressings

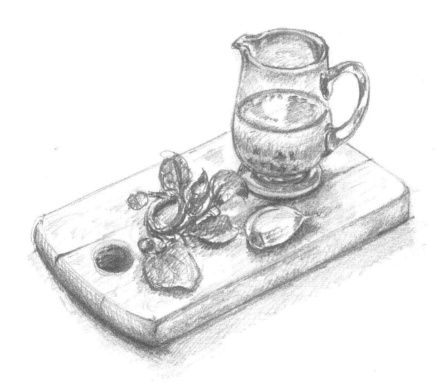

Oil and Lemon Dressing with garlic and herbs

When dining with guests, my salads are often an array of different salad vegetables arranged in heaps on a large shallow dish so that people can see what is what. This is accompanied with a separate dressing or two, and perhaps other savoury dishes and sauces. I usually make more than enough dressing for one meal so that there is something interesting to bring out of the fridge for the next meal or to put in a lunch box. Here are some 'vinaigrette' oil-and-vinegar-type dressings, made with fresh lemon juice instead of overly acidic vinegar, and some rich mayonnaise dressings. There are several delicious dressings made with almonds by different methods. You can use these methods with different nuts and seeds. You will also find some more adventurous dressings.

Oil and Lemon Dressing

If you want to be on a more alkaline diet, and still to have an acidic taste in your salads, it is time to say goodbye to balsamic vinegar, or any other kind of vinegar, and to say hello to lemon juice.

You can make a simple French-style dressing with oil and fresh lemon juice. Two thirds cold pressed oil to one third lemon suits many tastes, or try with oil and a mixture of lemon juice and filtered water if it is too strongly lemony.

Olive oil and walnut oil are traditional, and you can experiment with hazelnut oil and hemp oil. Season with finely chopped herbs, crushed garlic, mustard or tamari, as you will. Make it interesting by adding some very finely chopped mild onions, spring onions, chives, capers or olives.

Or, you can simply put out a little jug of lemon juice alongside a bottle or little jug of oil and let people work things out for themselves. Always use cold pressed organic oils. If you know everyone likes their salad dressed, and know it will all be eaten straight away, mix up your dressing to taste, pour it over your big green or mixed salad and turn gently with salad servers just before serving. One tradition is to cut a garlic clove and to rub it round the salad bowl before putting the salad leaves in the bowl.

....

Hippocrates House Dressing

This is the wonderful dressing that is always on the buffet at Hippocrates, and very much appreciated. It keeps well and you might want to make it in bigger quantities.

1 cup high quality cold pressed oil such as extra virgin olive, sesame, pumpkin, flax, hemp or walnut oil	2 cloves of garlic
	2 teaspoons ground mustard seed
2 ½ tablespoons fresh lemon juice	¼ teaspoon cayenne pepper
2 ½ tablespoons tamari	

Combine all the ingredients in a blender, adding 2-4 tablespoons of filtered water as you blend.

....

Almond or Tahini Ranch Dressing (Protein rich)

These are my favourite ever dressings for any raw sprouts and vegetables. They are quick and simple to make without any gadgets and it keeps well in the fridge.

Mix almond butter or tahini and unpasteurised sweet miso, three parts to one. Stir them together with just a hint of crushed garlic, and enough filtered water to make a pourable sauce.

Pour the ranch dressing over sprouts and vegetables for a delicious and simple meal or to take with you in your lunch box.

Thinned down, and with a little more garlic, other spices as you wish and perhaps more tamari, you can stir it through very fine 'angel hair' raw sweet potato noodles.

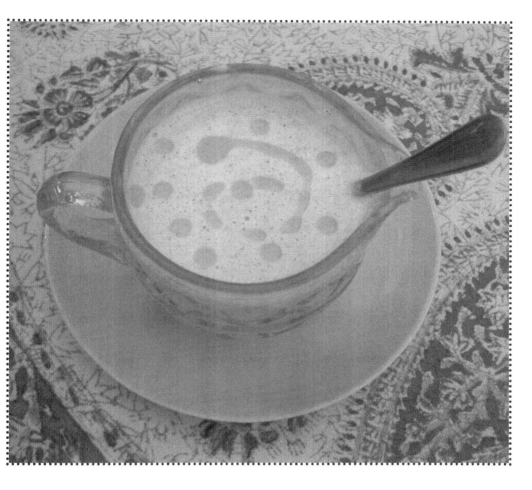

Almond Ranch dressing with an olive oil garnish

Curry Dressing

Here is one of a myriad possible variations on the oil-and-lemon-juice salad dressing theme.

Make an oil and lemon dressing and season it with a little curry powder, crushed garlic and a splash of tamari.

· ·

Japanese Style Dressing

Do Japanese people make dressings like this? As these ingredients are common in Japanese meals, why not? Perhaps they will as they get into this kind of fresh food.

¼ cup cold pressed sesame oil	torn shreds of dried sea
2 tablespoons lemon juice	vegetable
1 clove of garlic	A pinch of wasabi (Japanese
Optional: a tiny spoon/or drop	horseradish) powder or 1
of pure stevia extract, or ½	teaspoon prepared wasabi paste
teaspoon of honey or yacon	1 tablespoon soaked sesame
syrup.	seeds
1 tablespoon of tamari	¼ cup filtered water
I tablespoon seaweed flakes or	

Crush the garlic. Use the soaked sesame seeds or pulse them for a second in a grinder or blender to break them but still leave a rough texture. Mix all the ingredients together with a fork and add a little water till you get the right degree of lemon acidity. Season further as you wish, and serve with green salad and finely sliced radishes, perhaps with **Nori Rolls**.

Lemonnaise
(Protein rich)

This is similar to the ranch dressing but with garlic, lemon and mustard. It comes quite close to a traditional mayonnaise. This is easy and good with salad or as a dip with vegetable sticks.

One heaped tablespoon of almond butter
½ a lemon – all the skin, pith and juice but minus the pips, chopped
½ a cup of filtered water
A pinch each of mustard powder and cayenne pepper
A tiny piece of garlic
Optional: a splash of tamari or a pinch of sea salt

Blend all together.

....

Almond Mayonnaise
(Protein rich)

Another almond dressing – you can tell how much I like these and how often I make them! You can make this with the skins still on the almonds, and it is quicker that way, but for a smoother, whiter mayonnaise, you can 'blanch' the almonds. Settle down to a conversation with a friend or to something on the radio, and rub the skins off the almonds one at a time. The soaking should have loosened the skins so that they slip off easily.

1 cup almonds – soaked overnight, rinsed and drained
1 cup filtered water
½ a lemon – all the juice and a peeling of the skin
2 tablespoons cold pressed hemp oil
A pinch of cayenne pepper
Optional: a pinch of herb sea salt or a splash of tamari
Optional: 1 level teaspoon honey, or a tiny spoon or drop of pure
    stevia extract

Blend all together.

....

Almond Milk Mayonnaise
(Protein rich)

This is smooth and light, and not oily. All the oil is from the avocado
and the almonds, but you could add oil for a richer mayonnaise.

1 cup almonds, soaked over night, rinsed and drained
1 cup of filtered water
½ an avocado
Optional: a very tiny pinch of black Himalayan salt (for the egg taste)
Optional: a pinch of sea salt or a splash of tamari
¼ cup lemon juice
A few white mustard seeds or a small spoonful of mild prepared
    mustard
1 teaspoon honey/agave syrup/yacon syrup, or a tiny spoon or drop of
    pure stevia extract

Blend the almonds and water to a smooth cream. Squeeze through a juicing bag or put through a juicer on the appropriate setting for making nut milk. Blend the milk with the other ingredients and adjust seasonings to taste.

....

Lime and Walnut Mayonnaise (Protein rich)

This interesting dressing is best made from walnuts in their shells when you have just cracked open the shells and tasted them so that you know they are in their prime. Still soak them and rinse them to bring them back to life though.

1 teaspoon grated lime zest
The juice of a lime
1 tiny pinch of black Himalayan salt (for the egg taste)
Optional: a splash of tamari or a pinch of sea salt.
¾ cup cold pressed walnut oil
1 cup soaked and well rinsed walnuts
A small piece of garlic
Optional: 2 teaspoons honey/agave syrup or a tiny spoon or drop of
  pure stevia extract

Blend everything at high speed in a powerful blender. You can use any blender or processor, but for an ultra smooth texture a powerful one gives the best results.

Hot Sour Walnut Oil Dressing

This is an exceptionally nice complex rich-tasting sauce for a raw-stir or a salad, good enough to impress discerning diners, which most of us are. The walnut oil taste works well, but sesame oil would be good too.

A small bunch of coriander
The juice of a lime
1 teaspoon turmeric
½-1 clove of garlic
1 Brazil nut-sized piece of fresh ginger
4 tablespoons raw cold pressed walnut oil
Optional: 1 teaspoon honey or a tiny spoon or drop of pure stevia
   extract
1 teaspoon umeboshi paste or an umeboshi plum (Japanese salted
   plum) minus the stone
6 tablespoons filtered water

Blitz everything in a blender, adding more water little by little as necessary. The umeboshi paste should make it quite salty enough, and adds an interesting taste. That small quantity of plum should not be a food-combining issue.

Italian Mild Red Pepper Dressing

Here is another recipe that has rich red Italian flavour, but avoids the acid nature of tomatoes. Serve with salads and sprouts, and perhaps with dehydrated crackers that have plenty of herbs in them.

1 large clove of garlic
2 red capsicums or sweet red peppers
3 tablespoons cold pressed olive oil
2 tablespoons lemon juice
Optional: 1 tablespoon tamari
Filtered water as necessary
A handful of finely chopped fresh herbs such as basil, parsley and
  oregano

Blend everything together and adjust seasonings to taste. If you have a regular blender the dressing will have a rougher texture but will still taste good.

....

Carrot and Coriander Dressing

Carrot and coriander work together just as well in salad dressing as they do in soup, and I make this light dressing time and again. Use a food processor or a grinder rather than a high power blender, so that the herbs and carrot are still present in a grainy texture. Or, use your blender and go in short pulses on the slowest setting.

A medium-sized carrot

A small bunch of coriander

2 tablespoons cold pressed olive oil

4 tablespoons filtered water

A small piece of garlic

A splash of tamari or ¼ teaspoon sea salt or herb salt

The juice of half a lemon

Process all together except half the water. Then add the rest of the filtered water as needed and adjust the seasonings. Process till there are no large pieces of carrot present, but stop while it is still a mixture of carrot grains and herb flecks in a liquid dressing. Serve with very fresh light salad vegetables such as sunflower greens, pea greens, buckwheat lettuce, lettuce, cucumber, and red capsicum so that the experience is quite thirst quenching.

Good Salads

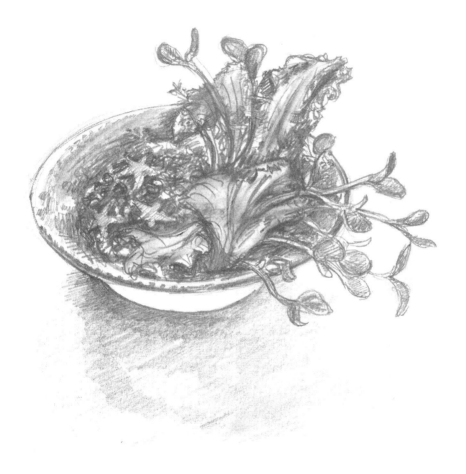

Lettuce, sunflower greens, and
a sprout salad with carrot stars

Be imaginative with salads. The colours, combinations of ingredients, and how you cut them make all the difference. You can combine many different vegetables or select two or three. You can serve dressings alongside or mix them in beforehand. Here are some suggestions:

- ❧ Chop or thinly slice cucumber. Slice it on the diagonal or cut it into small thin batons or sticks
- ❧ Grate carrot very finely or coarsely, slice wafer-thin or make thin strips with a julienne cutter
- ❧ Tear lettuce leaves instead of chopping them. Apparently they wilt less quickly that way
- ❧ Chop several shitake mushrooms very finely and stir into the dressing to marinate before mixing the dressing through the salad
- ❧ Soak some pecan nuts and slice them thinly before mixing them into the salad
- ❧ Add small, whole radishes to a finely sliced coleslaw
- ❧ For a very sunny salad, mix grated carrot, thinly sliced orange capsicum and finely sliced yellow chard from a rainbow chard mixture, and garnish with marigold petals and nasturtiums
- ❧ Mix sliced dandelion leaves and finely sliced mild onion with sliced pitted olives and **Italian Mild Red Pepper Dressing**
- ❧ Mix sliced red radishes, grated beetroot and shredded red cabbage, and scatter with little carrot stars made with a tiny cutter from a cookshop
- ❧ Garnish with chopped chives and other herbs
- ❧ Keep back one ingredient and arrange it last as an edging round the salad bowl
- ❧ Mix typical ingredients from one country, such as Chinese bean sprouts, finely sliced Chinese cabbage, finely sliced spring onions, and finely sliced carrot leaves with a gingery dressing for a Chinese salad
- ❧ Look at salad photos in recipe books

Dressed salads make meals interesting, whether for parties, potluck meals, family meals or dining for two. Remember to eat plenty of salad. Ample roughage is important for digestion and the water in the vegetables is the best kind of hydration.

Avocado Salad

Make this when avocados are plentiful, ripe and inexpensive. In fact, only ever eat avocados when they are ripe. This goes for all fruits as an unripe fruit can ruin a recipe as well as giving your system a hard time.

Chop a few avocados into a bowl and mix with any of the mayonnaise recipes and a few finely chopped herbs. Chives would be particularly good, or chives and a little mint.

....

Cucumber Salad

This is another salad that features a single vegetable. Slice a large cucumber as thinly as you can, perhaps cutting lengthwise strips out of the skin first so that you get a pattern when you slice across. Add a little very finely chopped mild onion, a little cold pressed olive oil, a squeeze of lemon juice and perhaps a splash of tamari, and mix gently. Under-season to feature the cucumber. Serve sprinkled with very finely chopped parsley.

Grated Carrot and Herb Salad

This is so simple that you do not need a proper recipe.

Grate a salad bowl full of carrot. Add plenty of chopped fresh herbs, perhaps from your garden. These might include chives, thyme, parsley, oregano and basil. Add a crushed clove of garlic and dress with good strong-tasting cold pressed olive oil and lemon juice. Season with little or no tamari. You may need to add a little filtered water, especially with large carrots that can be more dry.

....

Light Sunflower Greens Salad

These are the greens you can grow yourself to about 6 in/14 cm tall, with 2 seed leaves at the top of each stalk.

2 cups sunflower greens
2 cups finely chopped green lettuce
1 chopped firm but ripe avocado

Make a dressing of:

2 tablespoons unpasteurised sweet miso	A pinch of cayenne pepper
½ cup sea salad, nori, dulse or karengo sea vegetable	2 teaspoons lemon or lime juice
½ cup filtered water	A handful of fresh coriander, chopped

Mix the miso, water, cayenne and lemon or lime juice well. Add the sea vegetables and leave to soften. Toss the dressing with the avocado, greens and herbs in a salad bowl and serve.

Waldorf Salad
(Protein rich)

Traditional Waldorf Salad usually includes walnuts, celery and apple in mayonnaise. For better food combining, mine has the sweetness of carrots instead of the apples. One friend declared it to be 'gourmet restaurant standard'. Nice friend.

You could use any of the almond mayonnaise recipes in this book, or the one below here. Serves 4 as a side salad

3 large sticks of celery
½ cup of walnuts that have been soaked, dehydrated and broken into small pieces
1 small-medium carrot
3 tablespoons white almond butter
1½ teaspoons Dijon or other prepared mustard, or a little mustard powder
Optional: 1 teaspoon honey/agave syrup, or a tiny spoon or drop of pure stevia extract
Optional: A splash of tamari
1½ tablespoons lemon juice
2-3 tablespoons filtered water

Slice the celery across thinly, grate the carrot and put the celery, walnuts and carrots in a bowl. Mix the other ingredients together, and adjust the seasonings. Stir into the vegetables and serve.

Carrot and Red Lentil Salad with Beetroot Stars

This simple salad vanishes fast at raw potluck meetings! It enlivens a very green meal and the (optional) stars are easy to make if you can find a tiny star cutter in a cookshop. It is good, light and cheap and the lentils give you plenty of energy. Use red lentil sprouts that you have grown yourself and sprouted just till very short tails are developing. They look brown because they still have their skins, but you can see the red peeking through as they sprout. Start the sprouts 2 – 3 days in advance. When they are just right put them in the fridge until you make the dish, so they do not grow too much.

2 cups grated carrot
2 cups sprouted red lentils
4 teaspoons cold pressed olive oil
Optional: 2 teaspoons tamari
¼ teaspoon freshly ground cumin
A light grating of fresh ginger
Very thin beetroot slices for the decoration

Mix all the ingredients in a salad bowl. Go easy with the seasonings as this is intended as a very mild dish that is in contrast to stronger tastes in the meal. You can leave the oil out if you wish.

To decorate, cut very thin slices of beetroot. Rinse off the excess red colour and dry them on kitchen paper. Cut out tiny stars with a cutter or cut little diamonds with a knife and scatter them over the salad.

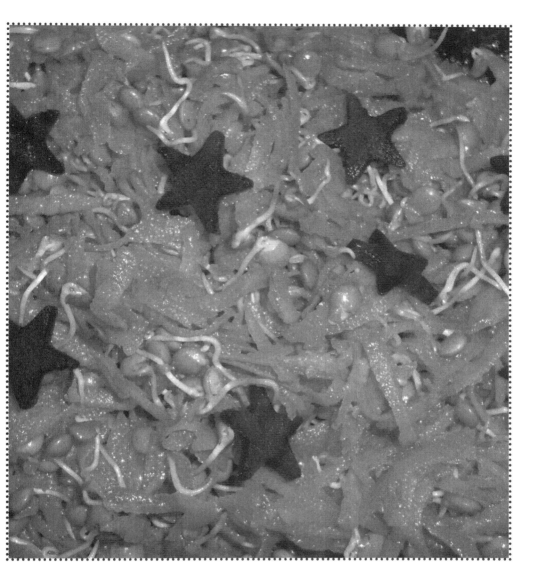

Carrot and Red Lentil Salad with beetroot stars

Green Lentil Salad

This is another good lentil dish, a reminder that simple and easy dishes are good. It is hardly even a recipe. You just mix plenty of sprouted lentils with a little very finely chopped mild onion, finely chopped red capsicum or sweet pointed pepper and finely chopped celery. Then you add a little cold pressed hemp or olive oil and season very lightly with tamari. Or, you can leave the salty seasoning out and appreciate the saltiness of the finely chopped celery.

Serve it as a salad in its own right or use in raw wraps, boats or tacos as the 'meat'.

....

Avocado and Hemp Seed Salad (Protein rich)

This is an oily mixture to use in small quantities as a filling in wraps, boats or tacos or with lighter salad dishes. Serves 4 as a side dish

2 teaspoons cold pressed olive oil
2 teaspoons lemon juice
¼ cup of tightly packed sliced or torn dried dulse, nori, karengo or 'salad mix' sea vegetables

1 tablespoon hulled hemp seeds
Optional: 2 teaspoons tamari
2 large chopped ripe avocados
2 tablespoons filtered water

Mix the oil, lemon, seaweed, hemp seeds and tamari and leave to soak, adding a little water if necessary. Chop the avocado and mix gently into the hempseed mixture.

As an alternative, halve the avocados and fill with the hempseed mixture, perhaps adding more hempseeds to thicken it.

You could also change the name and add finely sliced shitaki mushrooms with more of the dressing ingredients.

••

Sea Salad

This salad features sea vegetables, with their whiff of ozone sea breezes and their mineral salt tang. The carrot adds sweetness and a contrast of colour. The oil brings richness and the seasoning is only there to bring out the best in the sea vegetables.

1 cup grated carrot
1 cup 'sea salad', dulse or other light sea vegetables
1 cup filtered water
Optional: A splash of tamari
The juice of half a lemon
2 tablespoons cold pressed olive or sesame oil

Soak the sea vegetables in the water, chopping them up first if the pieces are very large. When they have absorbed plenty of water mix them with the grated carrot, half the lemon juice and the oil. Then, if you wish, season with just a touch of tamari, and perhaps more lemon juice.

Wasabi Salad

Wasabi is the pungent Japanese horseradish paste served with nori rolls. It meets seaweed in a different way in this salad, and they get on very well. Per person:

A large handful each of sunflower and snow pea greens
A small handful of dulse or karengo
I tablespoon finely chopped mild onion
2 teaspoons each of lemon juice and cold pressed sesame oil
1 tablespoon of filtered water
A small squeeze of all-natural wasabi paste
Optional garnish: **Tastied Sesame Seeds** or soaked sesame seeds

Mix the lemon, oil, water and wasabi together. Go easy on the wasabi unless you know the tastes of your diners well. You can always serve some separately for those who like it stronger. Rip the dulse or karengo into small pieces and mix with the salad and dressing in a serving bowl. Sprinkle with **Tastied Sesame Seeds** or soaked sesame seeds to garnish.

....

Mythical Island Salad
(Protein rich)

On a mythical island, somewhere in the South Seas between Japan and Korea, this is the kind of raw lunch they whip up in a hurry.

For each person:

2 large handfuls of any fresh sprouts and tray-grown greens
2-3 tablespoons of **Kim Chi,** preferably home made
Optional: a dash of tamari
½ an avocado, chopped
I tablespoon cold pressed sesame oil
2 sheets of untoasted nori sea vegetable
A chunk of cucumber, thinly sliced
A tablespoon of **Tastied Sesame Seeds**
A squeeze of lemon juice

Rip up the nori into small pieces and mix it with everything else and serve. Then, of course, the islanders chew mindfully before getting back to work.

....

Sweet Lemon Lettuce

This is an unusual sweet-sour salad with no sugary anything, just pure stevia extract. You would not guess though. The flavours could have come straight from a sweet shop.

2 tablespoons cold pressed olive oil
2 tablespoons lemon juice
Optional: a splash of tamari or a pinch of sea salt
I tablespoon cold pressed olive oil
A pinch of cayenne pepper and a tiny spoon or drop of pure stevia
  extract

Beat everything together with a fork and pour over ripped lettuce leaves and/or other light salad greens such as lambs' lettuce or buckwheat lettuce. Sweet lemon lettuce goes well next to other salads because the sweet-sour combination is quite a surprise.

Beansprout and Cucumber Salad with a Parsley, Carrot and Almond Dressing
(Protein rich)

Always include the skin of a cucumber, unless it is a bitter or tough-skinned variety. I am assuming organic cucumbers of course, but then I am assuming ALL organic produce in your kitchen, so that your food is as beneficial to you as possible!

2 cups of home-grown mung bean sprouts or 3 cups of purchased
   Chinese bean sprouts
2 cups finely chopped cucumber
¾ cup soaked almonds
1 small bunch of parsley
1 small clove of garlic
Optional: 2 teaspoons of tamari
1 small to medium carrot
The juice of half a lemon
Filtered water as needed

Using a processor rather than a blender, process the almonds to a sandy consistency. Add the garlic, chopped carrot and parsley, and continue. Add the lemon juice and tamari and a little water, and blend to a thin cream that still has the distinct grainy texture of the nuts, parsley and carrot. Stir into the bean sprouts and cucumber and serve.

Curry Salad
(Protein rich)

This is a finely chopped salad with a light curry dressing mixed through it. The soaked or sprouted sunflower seeds make it quite substantial. Instead of the individual spices you could experiment with different curry spices or mixed curry powders. Use less than you would if you were cooking the powders because flavour is not lost in the raw process.

Chop and mix together all of these:

1 perfectly, not overly, ripe avocado
½ a large cucumber, chopped
1 sweet pointed red pepper or red capsicum, chopped
½ cup lentil sprouts
½ a small mild onion, finely chopped
A small handful each of basil and coriander
½ cup sunflower seeds, soaked, or soaked and sprouted for two days
Season with:
1 tablespoon cold pressed olive oil
Optional: 1 tablespoon tamari
1 level teaspoon cumin powder
¼ level teaspoon cayenne powder (more if you want it quite hot)
¼ teaspoon powdered ginger
1 small clove of garlic, crushed

Mix the salad in a serving bowl and leave at room temperature before serving.

Beetroot Salad

I first made this to accompany a Thai meal, hence the basil and cayenne pepper, but it would work well with different meals if you go lightly with the cayenne or leave it out.

A good-sized bunch of beetroot or at least 1lb/500g
A small bunch of basil
A small clove of garlic
1 tablespoon cold pressed sesame oil
A pinch, or more to taste, of cayenne pepper
1 tablespoon lemon juice
A small piece of peeled fresh ginger
Optional: a splash of tamari

Squeeze, chop very finely or crush the garlic and ginger. Add to the washed, peeled and roughly chopped beetroot in a food processor. Add the pinch of cayenne, the washed basil leaves, lemon juice and a splash of tamari. Process until the beetroot is in tiny pieces like fine coleslaw, but not turning into a sauce.

Put everything a bowl. Adjust seasonings as you will and leave at room temperature for the flavours to mingle and develop before serving.

Thai Cucumber and Radish Noodle Salad

This salad with the joy of raw 'noodles' is the kind of food that gives raw vegan food a good name. It is a light dish that you could serve along with something richer such as an avocado salad. See the **Good Equipment** Chapter for how to make the noodles. The red radishes look good, but you could use some long white daikon radish instead.

1 cucumber

1 bunch of red radishes, the larger the individual radishes the better (Save any leaves to put in your green juice)

½ cup sesame seeds that have been sprouted, or left to soak for an hour, and rinsed.

1 tablespoon lemon or lime juice.

1 pinch cayenne pepper.

Optional: a tiny spoon or drop of pure stevia extract or half a teaspoon of honey/agave/yacon syrup

Optional: a splash of tamari

A handful each of basil and coriander leaves and a couple of sprigs of mint, all finely sliced.

½ sweet red pepper or red capsicum, finely sliced.

Turn the cucumber into long strands with a spiral pasta/noodle maker (coarse blade) and do the same with the radishes (medium blade). Put these noodles into a large bowl and stir in the other ingredients. Adjust the seasonings – perhaps adding a little more cayenne for authentic Thai heat. The touch of sweetness is a nod towards sweet and sour Thai tastes but the dish is also good without it and there is sweetness in the red pepper anyway.

Thai Coleslaw

This is a light, non-oily salad with a fiery touch. It is a good accompaniment to other raw oriental dishes. You might be noticing that I love Thai food. The bright flavours translate very well into raw dishes.

½ a large Chinese cabbage, sliced very finely
The juice of half a lime and a very little zest
A tablespoon each of finely chopped basil and coriander leaves
A pinch of cayenne pepper
Optional: 1 teaspoon honey or agave syrup or a tiny spoon or drop of
  pure stevia extract
1 grated carrot
½ teaspoon finely grated ginger
A splash of filtered water.

Mix all together and leave for the flavours to mix. This is a refreshing dish that is good without any salty seasoning.

Good Patés, Spreads

and Side Dishes

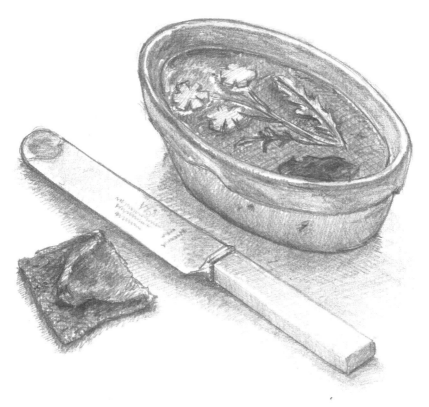

French Delicatessen Paté

Patés make good, solid centerpieces for meals and you can have fun decorating them. It seems to make them taste better. They keep well in the fridge and it is pleasing to find some left next day for making lunch.

The spreads include raw 'butters' that are comfortingly familiar on dehydrated crackers and breads, and excellent as spreads for lettuce, cabbage and seaweed wraps. If you include some cooked food in your life, they are good on steamed vegetables.

The side dishes are chunky relishes and other quite intense or solid dishes that are good accompaniments to salads and lighter dishes.

White Almond Paté
(Protein rich)

The point of this paté is to have it as a creamy foil to tasty dehydrated crackers and as a mild-flavoured dish for dipping vegetable sticks. By adding a little water you can turn it into a good 'sour cream' for raw tacos and nachos.

1 cup almonds soaked for a day or over night, rinsed and drained
1 small courgette, peeled
½ an avocado
A pinch each of powdered cloves, cinnamon and freshly grated nutmeg
A tiny piece of garlic
2 tablespoons of cold pressed hemp or mild-flavoured olive oil
The juice of half a small lemon
Optional: ¼ teaspoon sea salt or a splash of tamari
Filtered water

Rinse and drain the soaked almonds, and rub their skins off with your fingers. You could, of course, make this easier by pouring boiling water over them. I do not because I want them as raw as possible. Rubbing the skins off is not essential but the paté looks good white and would be smoother.

Blend or process everything except the avocado, adding water a teaspoon at a time until it is a thick not quite smooth cream. Blend in the avocados and leave it to sit for a while for the flavours to develop. It should be mild and creamy with a grainy texture, and the almond flavour coming through.

Simple Cucumber Paté
(Protein rich)

This is a gentle creation, almost like a butter. It is a good balance for more highly seasoned dishes and it is just right with vegetable sticks.

Use leftover minced cucumber fibres from juicing so that it is relatively dry.

1 cup minced cucumber fibres	1 level tablespoon sweet miso
1 cup ground almonds	Filtered water

Stir everything together, adding water as necessary to mix, but keeping the mixture quite stiff. Pat down into a suitable small dish and serve.

Sage and Thyme
Sunflower Paté (Protein rich)

When I make this one I am told it tastes like traditional paté. You can make it either in a food processor or in an auger juicer set up for mincing foods or making pasta. Put it through the juicer a second time for a finer paté.

2 teaspoons each dried sage and thyme, or twice as much chopped fresh	2 cups sunflower seeds, soaked for six or more hours
	4 tablespoons cold pressed olive oil

| 1 – 2 tablespoons tamari | Just enough filtered water to |
| 1 clove of garlic | process |

Drain the sunflower seeds and process with the oil, herbs, garlic and a tablespoon of the tamari. Add more tamari to taste, and only if absolutely necessary add a little water to process to paté consistency. Put the mixture into a serving dish and smooth the surface.

Serve with vegetable sticks or dehydrated crackers, or in wraps.

Almond and Whole Lentil Paté (Protein rich)

This recipe uses the almond fibre from making almond milk. Mixed with the whole sprouted lentils, it gives an interesting texture. The almond taste is delicious.

4 teaspoons sweet white or	Almond fibre from 1 cup
sweet brown miso	almonds for making milk
I tablespoon cold pressed olive	I cup green lentils barely starting
oil	to sprout
	A little almond milk

Soak the almonds overnight or all day and blend them with two cups of filtered water. Pour the mixture into a net bag to make the almond milk and put the fibre into a bowl. Do not squeeze every drop of milk out of the fibre. Mix the miso, tamari and oil with the almond fibre. Stir in the lentils and add a little of the almond milk if the mixture is too dry. Pat it into a serving dish. It should just about hold together.

This is also good with a touch of spice such as ground cumin or coriander seeds.

Light Paté of Celeriac and Courgette

These two vegetables are ones I would never have imagined would be nice raw.

1 cup chopped celeriac	A pinch of cayenne pepper
1 cup chopped courgette	1 level teaspoon of paprika
4 teaspoons of sweet miso	
1 tablespoon cold pressed olive oil	

Process the vegetables to rough paté consistency and mix with the miso, oil and cayenne pepper. Adjust the seasonings and press the mixture into a serving dish. Garnish with a dusting of paprika for contrast.

French Delicatessen Paté

When I worked as an au pair in Paris, cooking for a family of seven, I loved the traditional up-market delicatessens because everything was so exquisitely beautiful. Apparently, when the court chefs fled the palace in the French Revolution they set up delicatessens all over France and continued making court-quality delicacies. Paris patés are presented elaborately decorated with vegetable pieces in patterns and flower arrangements.

This is my version of a savoury paté with a translucent olive oil glaze misted over a decoration.

1 or 2 recipes of seed or nut paté, such as sage and thyme sunflower
  paté, made with minimal water so that it is relatively stiff, like a
  traditional paté.
2 tablespoons of cold pressed olive oil.

Pat the paté mixture down into an attractive serving dish.
Decorate the surface of the paté with very thin carrot slices cut into
flowers and with basil or flat parsley leaves, pressing them down lightly,
flush with the paté.

Pour the oil over the top to completely cover the surface, brushing it
gently over the decorations. You can put the finished paté in the freezer
for a little while to chill the oil enough to set it. It will go cloudy, but
you will still see the decoration through it.

Leave it to set in the fridge for a few hours. Serve at the last minute
as a centerpiece with raw breads or crackers, vegetable sticks or salad.

Olive, Almond and Cucumber Tapenade
(Protein rich)

Tapenade is usually an intensely salty olive paté. This development on
from the tradition is still rich and oily, but not so salty. The quantities
are vague because the cucumber part is the leftover fibres from juicing
cucumber. How dry the fibre is depends on your make of juicer, so guess
at this to get a mixture that you like.

1 cup or more cucumber solids from juicing cucumber

10-20 kalamata olives, depending on how salty and what size. You can use more if they are not very salty, or if you soak them overnight first

2 'dollops' (my mother's technical term), in other words two heaped tablespoons, of almond butter, preferably white almond butter

2 tablespoons cold pressed olive oil + more to garnish

Grind or blend the olives in the oil to a rough paste. Stir the olive paste into 1 cup cucumber solids and add the almond butter. Taste, and add more cucumber if you wish. Serve in a small dish drizzled with oil. Serve with crackers or as a spread on lettuce leaves. Spread on large basil leaves as a canapé.

••

Pineapple and Avocado Chutney

This is not brilliant food combining I admit, but the pineapple is particularly rich in enzymes. You only have a small amount so it is not a digestive disaster, but skip this one if you want to follow food combining precisely. Serves 4 as an accompaniment to a curry.

1 very thick slice of a large pineapple, chopped finely

The juice of half a lime

½ a large or 1 medium perfectly ripe, not squashy, avocado, chopped finely to match the pineapple

¼ teaspoon cayenne pepper

½ teaspoon curry powder

1 very small mild onion, chopped finely

2 teaspoons cold pressed sesame or olive oil

Optional: a pinch of sea salt or a splash of tamari

Stir everything together in a suitable serving bowl and leave for the flavours to develop. Serve at room temperature.

....

Sweet Ginger Relish

Grate a small lump of peeled fresh ginger and a carrot on a fine grater and mix them together. Add more grated ginger or carrot to get the balance of heat and sweetness that you like, and perhaps a squeeze of lemon juice. This is a good condiment with nori rolls and other Japanese-tasting food.

....

Cucumber Raita
(Protein rich)

Raita is a traditional accompaniment to a curry. This one is to accompany a raw, perhaps lightly dehydrated **Curry**. Instead of the usual yoghurt this raita has a nut cream and you can use any soaked nuts or seeds. I used almonds but walnuts, hazelnuts or sunflower seeds would be good too, or hulled hemp seeds. Add cayenne pepper if you wish.

½ – ¾ a large cucumber, chopped finely
The juice of ½ a lemon
½ a cup of filtered water
1/2 cup soaked nuts or seeds
Sprigs of coriander

Blend everything except the cucumber to a smooth cream, adding a little more water if necessary, and stir through the cucumber. I do not add any salt so that it is a good foil for the tamari taste in the curry. You could stir in finely chopped coriander and chopped mild onion, but plain cucumber is very good.

....

Cucumber Relish

Making green juice keeps leaving you with plenty of fibres. The cucumber fibres have a little juice and plenty of life left in them and I often wonder how to use them. They make a great relish.

Mix some fibres with a little lemon juice, oil, tamari and mustard, and cucumber juice if too dry.

To accompany a curry, add chopped coriander.

....

Radish Relish

This is a bright sauce that goes well with Japanese-style dishes. It also goes well with European-style foods such as the **Sweet Potato Wrapped Chipolatas**.

The juice of half a lemon
1 bunch of radishes
Optional: 1 teaspoon honey/agave syrup or a tiny spoon or drop of
  pure stevia extract
1 medium clove of garlic
4 tablespoons cold pressed sesame oil
2 tablespoons filtered water
3 Brazil nuts' worth of fresh ginger
Optional: a pinch of salt or a splash of tamari

In a powerful blender, blitz everything except half of the radishes and adjust the seasoning. If you use a regular blender or food processor you might want to grate the ginger finely first and leave out any stringy bits.

The next step is important to turn it into a relish, rather than into baby food. Add the radishes and pulse briefly until you have a grainy sauce flecked with the pink-red of the radishes.

....

Kim Chi

This is an easy version of Korean traditional spicy pickled vegetables. It is deliciously spicy and quite special for something that is so easy to make. The sea salt is to preserve it, but you can use the excess brine to season other dishes. Try it this way first, and then experiment with less salt.

I make mine in a special crock for kim chi and sauerkraut. It has two clay weights to hold down the vegetables and a china lid that sits in a rim of filtered water to keep out any stray bacteria of the wrong kind. You can also use Kilner jars.

1 Chinese cabbage, approximately a kilo or 2lbs, sliced so that the
   stalks are in roughly 1 inch/2 centimetre lengths
2 large carrots, coarsely grated
A bunch of red radishes, sliced across thinly
2 small-medium mild onions, sliced lengthwise into thin strips
I head of garlic and an equal amount of peeled ginger
2 teaspoons cayenne pepper, or grated fresh chili pepper to taste
I tablespoon sea salt
A good handful of dulse sea vegetable

Wash and slice the cabbage. Chop the dulse coarsely. Cut the root end off the head of garlic so that it is easy to peel each clove, and slice the peeled cloves. Grate the ginger finely. Grate the carrots coarsely. Put all the ingredients in a large bowl and stir together before putting them in your crock or jars. Weight them down in the crock or divide between the jars. Leave for several hours or overnight and check that sufficient juice has been released to cover the vegetables, easily reaching around the crock weights. You may have to push the vegetables down in the crock or jars so that the juice covers them. If there is still insufficient juice, add filtered water, ideally boiled and cooled first, to bring the liquid level just to the top of the pressed vegetables. Close up the Kilner jars. Put water round the rim of the crock to seal it and put the lid on. Keep in a cool place and leave for a week or so. Taste occasionally to check whether it is sufficiently soured. Kim chi keeps well in the fridge and the sour fermented taste matures interestingly over the days. The salty juice is delicious as a seasoning in salads and soups. Once you have made a successful batch, try with less or no salt and more seaweed.

....

Sauerkraut

Make this in the same way as **Kim Chi**, with finely sliced cabbage. You can add sliced onion and garlic, other vegetables, seaweed and/or herbs and spices such as dill and cumin. Use roughly the same proportions of salt and vegetables as with the Kim Chi. Once you have made a batch or two that works, try using using plenty of sea vegetables and spices instead of some or all of the salt to find a formula that works well for you. To spread the salt out, use the salty brine in different meals, perhaps in a soup or sauce.

Cucumber Spread
(Protein rich)

This is a dense spread, for example for cabbage or lettuce leaf wraps and boats. It is supposed to be quite plain for simple snacks or as a foil for creations that have more herbs or spices. It is another good way to use the cucumber fibres from juicing.

1 cup quite dry cucumber fibre from juicing
2 tablespoons tahini
2 tablespoons unpasteurised sweet miso
Filtered water to mix.

Mix the cucumber fibres, tahini and miso together. If too dry and thick, add a little water to make a stiffish paste. This spread is also good made with aged miso instead, in which case start with one tablespoon of miso and see how that tastes.

....

Avocado Butter

Mash or blend an avocado with a teaspoon of unpasteurised sweet miso. Taste, and add more miso if necessary, aiming at a mild taste with only a hint of saltiness – like butter! Or, just mash the avocado for sophisticated unsalted butter.

Nut Butter
(Protein rich)

Make your own raw butters from nuts and seeds you have soaked and dehydrated. Use a single auger juicer with the parts for making patés and pasta. To make sure you do not overheat the motor or block the juicer parts with solid nut, mix cold pressed oil with the nuts and seeds to soften the mixture.

Alternate a few nuts or seeds with oil, perhaps sesame or walnut oil, and watch that the mixture is moving right through.

Once you have made a rough butter you can put it back through the juicer to grind it further, but the end product is still likely to be more rough than bought nut butters. Try interesting mixtures such as sesame seeds, sesame oil and almonds.

....

Vegan Butter with Coconut Oil

This is a little like melted butter. The coconut butter taste makes a nice change but I would not have it all the time. Some say it is no better than cows' butter in health terms as it is a saturated fat.

6 tablespoons each cold pressed olive and coconut oils
A few drops of lemon juice
1 tablespoon of almond or other nut milk
Optional: a pinch of sea salt

Let the coconut butter soften at room temperature or on a warm windowsill. Mix everything together well and refrigerate until it sets, stirring again if necessary.

Miso and Olive Oil Butter

There are no nuts or seeds in this butter, so it would be good food combining with a carbohydrate meal of sprouted grain bread and salad.

4 tablespoons unpasteurised sweet miso
4 tablespoons cold pressed olive oil
2 teaspoons filtered water
2 teaspoons of lemon juice

Mix all the ingredients together to form an emulsion. Pour into a small dish and refrigerate overnight. If it does not set, put it in the freezer for a while to harden the olive oil more quickly, and put it back to the fridge. Serve straight from the fridge – it melts quickly!

Vary this with a little crushed garlic, or a little parsley chopped almost to a paste.

Butter Spread

As a butter fan I have made many attempts at a raw vegan version, and this is one of my best, so far. It is quite a runny butter that thickens a little in the fridge. For a thicker butter, add a little less water. Serve it on dehydrated crackers and breads, on sprouted Essene bread or over steamed vegetables.

½ cup good quality cold pressed oil, such as a mixture of walnut and
  sesame oil
½ cup filtered water
¼ cup ground chia seeds or Mila
1 tablespoon lemon juice
Optional: 1/4 teaspoon sea salt
A tiny pinch of turmeric for the butter colour

If you use chia seeds, grind them. Then blend everything together,
preferably in a powerful blender that can grind out any graininess in the
Mila/chia seeds.

You can vary the recipe by using different oils such as olive or
pumpkin, each of which will give it a different character. Blend in a little
garlic or add finely chopped herbs for garlic or herb butter.

Good Sauces, Dips and Pestos

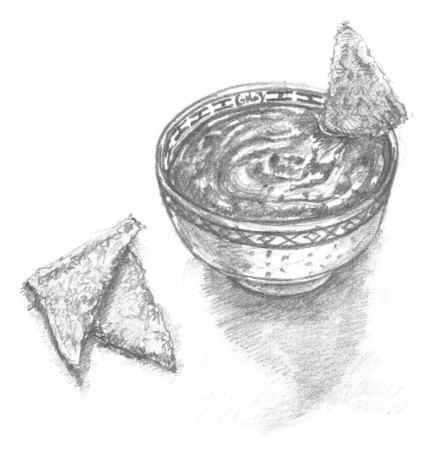

Avocado and Red Pepper Salsa with raw Corn Chips

Raw food does not mean only having conventional salads. These recipes will transform your meal repertoire and expand your imagination. They are good accompaniments to cooked food as well as raw. Try the raw sauces over steamed organic vegetables or vegetables that have been sliced thinly, mixed with a little good oil and dehydrated for a little while to wilt them..

Hollandaise Sauce
(Protein rich)

This is my version of the classic French sauce that is lovely over vegetables. Try it poured over courgettes and asparagus that have been brushed with a little oil and wilted in a dehydrator for an hour or so. The saffron is good if you have it, to impart an authentic pale yellow colour, but it is not essential for the taste.

1 cup walnuts, soaked overnight, drained and rinsed twice
½ cup cold pressed walnut oil
4 teaspoons of lemon juice
Optional: ½ teaspoon black Himalayan salt (for the egg taste)
A generous grating of nutmeg
4 teaspoons of filtered water
Optional: a pinch of saffron
Optional: a splash of tamari/ or a pinch of sea salt

Blend all together in a powerful blender for a few seconds on high speed. Leave it to sit for a few minutes to soften the saffron, and blend again to distribute the saffron colour.

Serve straight away or refrigerate and bring back to room temperature before serving.

Macadamia and Carrot Cheesy Sauce
(Protein rich)

This sauce is good with courgette pasta and in lettuce and cabbage wraps. It is good on a raw pizza or as a raw lasagne layer, and it serves 4 over raw 'pasta'.

20 macadamia nuts, soaked
1 cup almond milk or other nut milk, preferably home-made
The juice of half a lemon
2 medium carrots
A pinch each of cayenne and mixed spice

A pinch of oregano or other dried herbs, or a few sprigs of fresh herbs
1 avocado
½ a clove of garlic
Optional: a splash of tamari

Blend or process the soaked macadamia nuts in the nut milk. Add the chopped carrot, lemon juice and garlic and blend or process till it is as smooth as possible. Add the seasonings and the avocado, and blend or process till thick and creamy.

Sunflower Sour Cream

Use this simply delicious cream as you would regular sour cream, in tacos and other Mexican dishes, in wraps or thinned a little and swirled into soup.

1 cup of sunflower seeds, soaked over night or all day
1 cup filtered water
4 teaspoons of lemon juice, or more to taste
¼ cup of cold pressed hemp oil

Blend everything together. This really does not need any seasoning and is good just like this as a foil for other flavours.

....

Chinese Lemon Sauce

This sweet and sour sauce is inspired by the one served in Chinese restaurants. I love it over Chinese vegetables, such as a mixture of Chinese beansprouts, Chinese cabbage, bok choy, radishes and spring onions.

For something more substantial, have it with lightly marinated **Tempeh Slices with Garlic** that have been warmed through and dried a little on the outside in your dehydrator.

Per serving:

½ teaspoon each of ground flax and ground chia seed/Mila
A pinch of cayenne pepper
2 tablespoons lemon juice
Garlic powder
The finely grated zest of ½ a lemon
A tiny spoon or drop of pure stevia extract, or 1-2 teaspoons of honey
  or agave syrup
Optional: a splash of tamari or a pinch of sea salt
1 tablespoon sesame oil or other good quality cold pressed oil
1 cup filtered water

Mix into a thin sauce and stir it through sprouts and plenty of finely-cut vegetables. To serve it warm, warm the vegetables and the sauce in the dehydrator first and use warm bowls for mixing and serving. Or, warm the sauce gently by stirring over a low heat with a clean finger and serve over tempeh slices warm from the dehydrator.

....

Carrot and Sesame Curry Sauce (Protein rich)

This sauce includes a tiny pinch of asafoetida, an eastern spice that adds a hint of something good, in a similar way to garlic but quite different. The Chinese name for it is *hing*. If you put in too much you may hate it, so I really do mean a tiny pinch. Asafoetida is good in any curry creation. The sauce is delicious without it, but if, like me, you enjoy exploring new tastes you might want to track some down and try it in other Indian dishes as well.

2 medium carrots, chopped
3 tablespoons thin raw white tahini
Half a lemon with the pips removed, chopped
¼ – ½ teaspoon cayenne pepper or a small piece of fresh red chili pepper
1 level teaspoon cumin seeds or powder
Optional: 1 pinch asafoetida/hing
Filtered water
Optional: a splash of tamari/or a pinch of sea salt

Blend or process all the ingredients except the salt or tamari and with only ¼ teaspoon cayenne pepper, adding just enough water to make a pouring sauce. Taste, and add a little sea salt or tamari and more cayenne if you wish.

This sauce is delicious over a mixture of sprouts. It has a real kick to it, or, if you prefer, a gentle nudge.

Sour Curry Sauce

This may not be a conventional curry sauce, but it is *hot*, robust, garlicky, sour and hits the taste buds from various angles. It is actually *hot*, as in going out for an Indian or Thai meal. The dried lemon or lime (I have seen it called both, but it is the same little dried citrus fruit) is an ingredient that perks up many dishes. See if you can find some in an oriental or Indian delicatessen. The taste is different from usual lemons/limes. Serves 4 over salad.

1 red capsicum or sweet red pepper
1 ripe lemon
Optional: a small slice of dried lemon/lime
2 cloves of garlic
A large pinch of cinnamon
1 level teaspoon cayenne pepper or a piece of fresh red chili pepper
2 tablespoons sesame seeds, soaked
4 tablespoons filtered water
Optional: splash of tamari or ¼ teaspoon sea salt

Blend all together and pour over a salad. For a Thai salad, include chopped coriander, spring onions, and basil.

It can be served in a jug as a separate hot sauce alongside other not-hot dishes for people to take if they wish. This kind of sauce keeps me on this way of eating!

Sauerkraut Sauce

I once had delicious fried German sauerkraut potato cakes with sauerkraut cooked into them and I was wondering what to do to create that soft potato and sauerkraut experience. Here is my creation, a simple blended sauce to serve over steamed sweet potatoes or grated courgettes and chopped avocado.

Add a big sprout salad and it is a complete meal. Because the sauerkraut is sour, the sauce works well as a dressing on the salad too.

With the beneficial micro-organisms from the sauerkraut, the miso and the tamari this is very helpful live food for intestinal health.

2 cups of drained unpasteurised sauerkraut
3 dessertspoons cold pressed olive oil
I tablespoon unpasteurised sweet miso
½ cup filtered water
Optional: 1 tablespoon tamari
I small clove of garlic

Blend all together. Adjust the seasonings by adding a little of the sour salty brine if really necessary (It should not be with all that miso and sauerkraut), or adding a little more oil for a richer sauce. Serve as it is or gently warmed, as usual stirring with a clean finger so as not to over-heat your unpasteurised sauce!

Thai Nut Butter Stir-Raw Sauce
(Protein rich)

6 tablespoons nut butter such as macadamia or pecan, or ¾ cup of
   whole nuts, soaked
¾ cup filtered water
1 – 2 tablespoons tamari
1 teaspoon honey/agave/yacon syrup, or a tiny spoon or drop of pure
   stevia extract
2 teaspoons lemon juice
2 large cloves of garlic
A pinch of cayenne pepper, or up to 1 teaspoon to taste
2 handfuls each of basil and coriander leaves.

Blend or process the ingredients together with half the water to a smooth cream. Pour into a bowl. Use the rest of the water to rinse out the processor or blender and stir into the sauce in the bowl. Adjust the seasonings and serve over an oriental mixture of vegetables such as Chinese mung bean sprouts, finely sliced Chinese cabbage leaves and spring onions, and sweet corn sliced straight off the cob.

Garnish with finely chopped red onion and basil and/or coriander.

Mild Pepper Sauce

Version 1 is smooth and mild, although you could spice it up with more cayenne and lemon juice if you wish. It is creamy from the avocado.

In Version 2 the focus is all on the red capsicums or sweet red peppers. Serves 4.

Version 1

A small piece of fresh red chili pepper or a large pinch of cayenne pepper	The juice of ½ a lemon
	4 tablespoons cold pressed sesame oil
½ a small mild onion	1 tablespoon of tamari
1 clove of garlic	2 cups of filtered water, less to start
2 red capsicums or sweet red pointed peppers	2 avocados

Blend everything together with half of the water until smooth. Adjust the seasonings, add more water as necessary, and serve over sprouts and finely sliced salad vegetables, perhaps with chopped coriander leaves.

Version 2

2 red capsicums or sweet red pointed peppers, roughly chopped	1 clove of garlic
	2 slices of mild onion
1 teaspoon lemon juice	Optional: 2 splashes of tamari

Blend all together, pushing the pepper chunks down in the blender and only adding a little filtered water if absolutely necessary. This is good mixed with chopped avocado and served in lettuce or cabbage wraps.

Red Pepper Ketchup

You need not feel deprived with this raw way of eating, and this ketchup is a good non-tomato sauce to have with dehydrated chipolatas or burgers, and to go in lettuce or cabbage wraps. It is concentrated and the idea is to have just a tablespoon or so per serving, as perhaps you *used to have* of that red stuff in a squeezy bottle.

4 large red capsicums or pointed red peppers	1 pinch cayenne pepper
2 tablespoons lemon juice	½ teaspoon each ground cinnamon and ground ginger
4 teaspoons of honey/agave/ yacon syrup or two tiny spoons or drops of pure stevia extract	Optional: 1 tablespoon tamari

Blend all together. Do not add any further seasoning because the flavours will concentrate. Pour the mixture into a large shallow dish and place in the dehydrator. Dehydrate to reduce the sauce for about an hour, stirring occasionally. Pour into a jug to serve.

Thai Hot Sauce

This is very fiery little sauce to serve alongside oriental salads and dishes such as the **Macadamia Stir-Raw**. Those who like it hot can drizzle a few drops over their food and pretend they are sitting outside a Singapore cafe in tropical heat.

2 teaspoons lemon juice	Optional: a splash of tamari or ½ teaspoon sea salt
2 teaspoons filtered water	

4 teaspoons sesame seeds, soaked or crushed	1 teaspoon cold pressed sesame oil
½ teaspoon honey or a tiny spoon of pure stevia extract	½ teaspoon cayenne pepper

Mix the ingredients together and leave for the flavours to develop, adding a little more water if you wish.

Serve in an egg cup sized bowl with a mustard spoon.

....

Indonesian Satay Sauce
(Protein rich)

This thick rich hot sauce takes me back to the Javanese street stalls in night markets where I first tasted all kinds of exotic spicy savoury Indonesian delights. The taste and texture of pine nuts or pecan nuts is a good alternative to peanuts (see the **Good Ingredients** section). Serve satay sauce with little sprouts in Chinese cabbage leaf wraps, as a dipping sauce with thin sticks of carrot, sweet red pepper, celery, cucumber and daikon radish, or with satay sticks – see **Indonesian Satay** in the **Good Savoury Dishes** section. You can also thin it with young coconut milk or filtered water and stir it through courgette noodles or a sprout salad.

1 ½ cups pine nuts or pecan nuts, or a mixture, soaked	Optional: a pinch of ground star anise
½ cup cold pressed sesame oil	4 teaspoons lemon juice
2 teaspoons paprika pepper	2-4 tablespoons tamari
½ teaspoon cayenne pepper or a small piece of fresh red chili pepper, or more to taste	2-3 teaspoons honey/agave syrup/yacon syrup, or a tiny spoon or drop or more of pure stevia extract
A small piece of garlic	

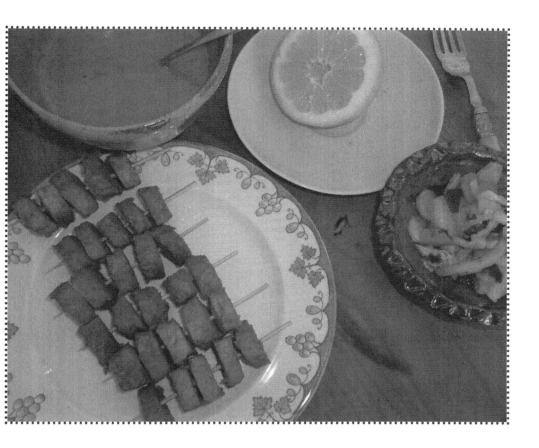

Indonesian Satay Sauce with Tempeh Satay,
kim chi and lemon

Blend the nuts for a few seconds until they are broken down but still have some texture. Take about half out of the blender and put them in a bowl. Add the rest of the ingredients to the blender and blend until smooth, adjusting the seasonings to taste. To be authentic it should be extremely hot from the cayenne or chili pepper, sweet and quite salty, but it never needs to be served in large quantities. Add the contents of the blender to the rest of the pine nuts in the bowl. Stir all together. To appreciate the tastes, serve at room temperature rather than from the fridge.

Miso Gravy

I was brought up on beautifully cooked meat-and-three-veg meals with the best of gravies, and I still love gravy. I perfected miso gravy in my pre-high-raw days and *had* to recreate it in raw. If you eat some cooked food, try this with delicately steamed vegetables and rice. For all-raw it is good with dehydrator–wilted vegetables and dehydrated burgers or chipolatas.

1 cup filtered water
3 tablespoons cold pressed olive oil
1 small pinch cayenne pepper
A very small piece of fresh ginger or a pinch of powder
2 teaspoons lemon juice

¼ small or ½ large Avocado
Optional: 1 tablespoon tamari
2 teaspoons unpasteurised aged miso
1 very small piece of garlic

Blend all together. Misos vary. Add a little more if it really is not salty enough for you, but hopefully in time you will want less and less salty tastes.

Ginger Gravy
(Protein rich)

This gravy is good with steamed vegetables or grains. It is quite a plain sauce with a little bite in the ginger.

2 Brazil nuts-worth of grated fresh ginger	1 small carrot
A pinch of cayenne pepper	½ cup soaked sunflower seeds
Optional: 4 teaspoons tamari	¾ cup filtered water

Blend everything together and adjust the seasonings to taste.

Avocado and Red Pepper Salsa

Dance around the kitchen as you magic up this spicy salsa. There is a chance you might all eat it up dipped in home made corn chips, before you even get to the dinner table.

1 large red capsicum pepper or 2 sweet pointed red peppers	A tiny piece of garlic
Optional: 1 tablespoon tamari	1 tablespoon lemon juice
Optional: ½ teaspoon cumin	1 tablespoon cold pressed olive oil
1 pinch of cayenne pepper, or more to taste	¼ – ½ small mild onion
	1 large perfectly ripe avocado

Blend everything except the avocado and onion in a food processor until grainy. Chop the avocado finely. Add about ¼ to the processor and pulse for a few seconds to thicken the mixture. Add the rest of the avocado and the onion chopped as finely as possible and process for a further 2 seconds only – to keep some texture.

Serve in a bowl with raw **Corn Chips**.

It is also lovely served in small spoonfuls in large basil leaves as a canapé.

....

Red Pepper Salsa

This is a good alternative to traditional tomato salsa. Follow the **Avocado and Red Pepper Salsa** recipe, only leave out the avocado and add an extra half a red capsicum or sweet red pepper. You could stir in a little finely chopped cucumber without the peel for texture, and make it more freshly fiery by blending in a little piece of fresh raw red chili pepper.

....

Guacamole

This is traditionally a raw dish. Just make a mixture of mashed avocados with a little lemon juice, crushed garlic, and perhaps a pinch of sea salt or splash of tamari. You can serve it lumpy or make it super-smooth in a food processor or blender, and you can heat it up with a little cayenne pepper or by blending in a tiny piece of fresh red chili pepper.

The Best Ever Pasta Sauce
(Protein rich)

This is to serve over freshly made 'courgetti' pasta or to use in a raw lasagne. It is a rich red Mediterranean-style sauce that steers clear of tomatoes. You could add a few chopped vine-ripened tomatoes, but it is delicious as it is. Serves 4

3 red capsicums or sweet red peppers
1 small red onion
2 generous handfuls of fresh basil
1 teaspoon dried mixed herbs or herbes Provençales, or a teaspoon each of finely chopped fresh oregano and thyme
About 16 pitted olives

½ cup pine nuts
½ teaspoon harissa powder or cayenne pepper
1 cup cold pressed olive oil
1 large clove of garlic
Optional: a splash of tamari and/or a pinch of sea salt and/or a squeeze of lemon juice

Blend the garlic, the chopped de-seeded capsicums and ½ a cup of the oil until smooth. A powerful blender is good. In an ordinary blender, crush the garlic first just in case.

Pour into a large bowl, leaving a little of the sauce behind in the blender. Add the pine nuts to the blender and blitz just for a couple of seconds. This should give you a mixture of finely chopped and larger chunks of pine nuts, with some left whole.

Scrape all of this into the large bowl. Chop the onions very finely. Slice the basil finely so you get fine strips. Cut the olives into fine slices. All this is better done by hand than in a processor to give interesting textures. Stir all these into the sauce in the bowl along with the rest of the olive oil. Season to taste and leave at room temperature for the flavours to develop. Serve with courgette pasta, allowing a courgette per person and an extra one, more for big appetites and for Italians!

Pesto
(Protein rich)

Traditional Italian pesto is a heavenly mixture of ground pine nuts, finely grated cheese, fresh basil, salt, pepper and crushed garlic, which can be stirred through pasta.

Years ago in Bali I tasted fresh cashew nut and coriander pesto, which set me off in all kinds of new pesto directions. Here is a raw vegan version of a traditional pesto, and also one I made earlier with what was to hand. The basic pesto taste and texture come from mixing ground nuts, with very finely chopped herbs, good quality cold pressed oil, crushed garlic, salt and a little lemon juice to give the sour edge that the cheese would have provided. Go ahead and try different combinations of nuts or seeds and herbs. Pumpkin seeds and thyme might be good.

As well as stirred through pasta, use pesto as a spread on a raw pizza and in wraps.

Traditional Pesto
(Protein rich)

This is the vegan version of the traditional Italian green pesto made with pine nuts. As I write, pine nuts are relatively expensive and so I would make this for a special occasion, or make it with sunflower seeds.

Serves 4 stirred into courgette pasta

¼ cup pine nuts and/or sunflower seeds soaked for a few hours
¼ cup water
The juice of a small lemon
Optional: pinches of sea salt or splashes of tamari
4 tablespoons finely chopped basil
1 large or 2 small cloves of garlic
¼ cup cold pressed oil
Optional: ½ a mild onion, very finely chopped

Grind the pine nuts/sunflower seeds lightly in a food processor and add the garlic, water, lemon juice and oil. Process to a smooth cream or a grainy cream, according to your tastes. Turn into a bowl and stir in the basil, onion if you wish, and season with a little sea salt or tamari.

For pesto pasta, make 'pasta' with 4-6 small-medium courgettes and stir the pesto in. Do this ahead of time if you can, so that the pasta softens and the flavours blend in well.

Parsley and Macadamia Nut Pesto
(Protein rich)

This is a pleasantly mild and creamy pesto. You can stir into courgette pasta and serve it along with a salad with contrasting bright colours and flavours. Serves 4.

2 tablespoons raw macadamia nut butter
4 tablespoons cold pressed olive oil
A handful of parsley
Optional: a pinch of sea salt
The juice of ½ a lemon
4-6 courgettes cut into raw 'pasta'

Chop the parsley very, very finely with a heavy cook's knife, holding the tip of the knife between your fingers and chopping down on the parsley with the other hand, till it is virtually a paste (otherwise you get rough pieces in a soft pasta dish). Stir other ingredients in and mix through the courgette 'pasta'.

Good
Savoury Dishes

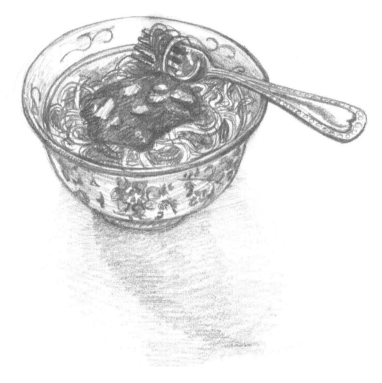

Raw Courgette Pasta with Best Ever Pasta Sauce
and Sunflower Pecorino Shards

These recipes are for substantial dishes for your raw meals. They have more in common with other traditional dishes than with traditional salads. Pair them with salads for meals with a good balance of tastes and textures: good square meals.

Curry and Biriani

This curry is made by wilting the vegetables in a dehydrator, and drying them a little, so that they have an interesting slightly oily texture on the outside, but are still moist. The flavours mix well. You can have a blended curry sauce, such as **Sour Curry Sauce** or **Carrot and Sesame Curry Sauce,** as part of the meal as well, perhaps creating a biriani by mixing this curry with some warmed courgette 'rice' and serving it with a curry sauce and a salad. You can vary the dish by using different curry powder blends or creating your own. I often use packets of interesting blends from Indian delicatessens, particularly Southern Indian varieties from their vegetarian cuisine.

½ small red or white cabbage
2 carrots
1 small red onion
1 cup finely chopped kale
1 corn garlic
1 Brazil nut-sized piece of ginger
2 teaspoons curry powder
2 teaspoons lemon juice
Optional: 1 tablespoon tamari
2 tablespoons cold pressed sesame or olive oil

Grate the carrots coarsely. Slice the cabbage and onion finely in a food processor or by hand with a sharp knife. Grate or crush the garlic and ginger finely. Mix the ingredients together in a bowl and spread thinly on dehydrator sheets.

Dehydrate for about 2 – 3 hours till limp but not dried out and serve warm straight from the dehydrator. You can completely dry out any leftovers and sprinkle them over another meal.

Comfort Pasta

This is simple, plain, satisfying, and easy to rustle up for one person, or for a crowd. It is the sort of food I like when I curl up with a book. Per person:

1 medium-large courgette	1 – 2 tablespoons cold pressed
A few finely chopped sliced	olive oil
olives	Optional: Sea salt to taste or
Optional: A little finely chopped	tamari
mild onion	

With a julienne cutter or a *Benriner* or similar, turn the courgette into pasta. Add the olives and, if you wish, the onion. The salt in the olives might be quite sufficient without adding any additional salt or tamari. Stir everything together and eat, perhaps while turning the pages of a good book such as this one.

. . . .

Orange Angel Hair Sweet Potato Pasta

I never considered eating sweet potatoes raw, but as fine pasta they are interesting. The texture improves if you leave the dish to sit for a while.

Turn a large sweet potato into very thin angel hair pasta with a *Benriner* or other device that will make very fine raw pasta.

Add:

A tablespoon of finely chopped herbs
A tablespoon of finely chopped spring onions
The juice of an orange (or, for better food combining, a little fine
  orange zest, a squeeze of lemon juice and half a cup of filtered
  water)
1 level teaspoon turmeric
A pinch of cayenne pepper
Optional: a splash of tamari or a pinch of sea salt
A tablespoon of cold pressed sesame oil

Mix everything together gently to avoid breaking the pasta. Leave to
marinate at room temperature and serve as a side dish.

....

Lettuce and Cabbage Wraps

These wraps are top in a new class of their own. They are good vehicles
for interesting mixtures of leftovers, and are easy food to eat at work or
when travelling.

Try:
- lettuce leaves 'buttered' with soft raw paté or dip, filled with
  sprouts, topped with soft dulse or karengo seaweeds and rolled up
  into wraps. Those wraps have a very nice balance as the dulse or
  karengo give a chewy bite, and the savour of the paté or dip and the
  seaweed are offset by the lettuce and sprouts. Try using just lentil
  sprouts, because sometimes it is good to appreciate a single type of
  sprout. Lentils are pleasantly sweet, but any sprouts would be good.
- lettuce leaves filled with a mixture of red pepper sauce and chopped
  avocado

- ✿ thin white or red cabbage leaves filled with paté, and sunflower and snow pea tray greens
- ✿ wrapping leftover raw creations in cabbage or lettuce leaves as a quick and easy lunch

....

Bacon, Lettuce and Sweet Red Pepper Wraps
(Protein rich)

Move on from BLT: these wraps are rich and delicious with an interesting mixture of tastes and textures, including marinated **Aubergine or Courgette Rashers** in the **Good Dehydrated Creations** section (only you do not have to dehydrate them). The delicious rashers are remarkably bacon-like. Some people raise health questions about aubergines (In the same family as tomatoes and potatoes) and may prefer to use courgettes.

Wraps

Soft round lettuce leaves or cos/romaine lettuce leaves.
Choose lettuce leaves that are a good shape for wraps. Put a handful of sprouts along the centre of a wrap and top with a slice or two of marinated 'bacon'. Spread a little sauce along the top and roll up. Repeat with all the ingredients.
Makes about a dozen good-sized wraps, or more small party canapés.

Filling

Plenty of sprouts of any kind and tray greens.

Red Pepper Sauce

1 cup sunflower seeds, soaked and, if possible, just beginning to sprout
1 sweet red pepper or red capsicum, chopped roughly
Optional: 1 tablespoon Braggs or Marigold Liquid Aminos, or tamari
1 medium clove of garlic
¼ teaspoon cayenne pepper
2 tablespoons lemon juice and a pinch of zest
1 tablespoon filtered water
¼ cup of cold pressed sesame oil
Blend the sauce ingredients together and adjust the seasonings.

....

Chinese Cabbage Boats

Chinese cabbage leaves and stalks are so fresh and crunchy that it would be a pity to wrap them round as you would a more limp cabbage leaf. That is why I call these boats. Instead, Cut the base off the Chinese cabbage so that you can easily pull off enough leaves for 3-4 per person. Pile them in a serving dish on the table and serve with a choice of sprouts, tray-grown greens, one or two dips, sauces, dressings or relishes and whatever else you have to hand. People assemble their own cargo in their boats. **Indonesian Satay Sauce** (Protein rich) goes particularly well with the crisp leaves.

Red Cabbage Rolls

Red cabbage has a deep vibrant purple colour that stands out on a table laden with green salad dishes, although you can use white cabbage if you prefer. The rolls are stuffed with a slightly Japanese filling.

1 red cabbage

A large handful of 'sea salad' seaweed or soft dulse torn or cut into small pieces

A thumb-sized piece of ginger, very finely grated

½ small mild onion, very finely chopped

Tamari to taste

A teaspoon of honey or agave syrup, or a tiny spoon or drop of pure stevia extract

½ cup of ground almonds or almond fibre from making almond milk

1 avocado, chopped finely

1 small-medium courgette grated

Wooden cocktail sticks

1 tablespoon filtered water

Grate the courgette and mix with the seaweed, onion, ginger and a tablespoon of water. Leave the seaweed to absorb the water and to soften. Add the honey/agave or stevia and the tamari and mix well. Add the ground almonds or almond fibre and mix again to a stuffing consistency. Adjust the seasoning to taste. Add a little more water if necessary, but make them too dry rather than too liquid, so that this is easy finger food. Fold in the avocado gently and leave all to thicken slightly.

Meanwhile, cut off the base of the cabbage so that you can easily peel away whole leaves. Cut each leaf in such a way that you have reasonably flat pieces without thick stalk. Save the stalks for making green juice. Add stuffing to each leaf piece. Roll the leaf up and secure with a cocktail stick. Depending on the size of your leaf pieces, this should make about 20 rolls.

Tabouleh

Traditional tabouleh is a mixture of kibbled wheat or couscous, both relatively acidic, with a great deal of finely chopped parsley and some chopped onion and tomato. I make tabouleh varieties so often that I have included three versions. You could, of course, make traditional tabouleh less acidic by substituting sweet red pepper for the tomato, and steamed millet (soaked overnight first) for the couscous, but here are my four raw versions:

1. Buckwheat Tabouleh (Carbohydrate rich)

This uses sprouted buckwheat as the grain.

Soak and sprout 2 cups of ordinary un-toasted and de-hulled buckwheat for a day or two, rinsing often and thoroughly, until it barely begins to sprout. Use the buckwheat as the 'grain' in this fairly traditional version:

½ cup very finely chopped parsley
½ cup finely chopped cucumber
2 tablespoons lemon juice
2 tablespoons cold pressed olive oil
¼ cup of finely chopped mild onion
1 finely chopped sweet red pepper or red capsicum pepper
Powdered sea vegetables or tamari to taste

Mix all together. These are very rough quantities. Work with what you have and season to taste. Add chopped olives if you wish, or serve some alongside with a green salad, oil and lemon dressing and perhaps a paté or dip with Mediterranean herbs such as thyme and oregano.

2. Sprouted Quinoa Tabouleh (Carbohydrate-Rich)

Make this in exactly the same way as the buckwheat tabouleh, using 2 cups of sprouted quinoa.

3. Courgette Tabouleh

Make this in exactly the same way but use 2 cups of grated courgettes instead of the buckwheat for the 'grain'. The courgettes take up the flavours well.

4. Almond Tabouleh (Protein rich)

When you make almond milk there is fibre left in the juice bag, still with some almond taste. This tabouleh uses the almond fibre in a very pleasant side dish.

Equal quantities of:

Leftover almond fibre from making almond milk
Cold pressed olive oil
De-hulled hemp seeds
Finely chopped parsley
Finely chopped red capsicum pepper
½ the quantity of finely chopped mild onion.

Mix all together and season lightly to taste with tamari and perhaps a squeeze of lemon juice. It is always better to under-season and to provide tamari at the table. That way everybody is happy.

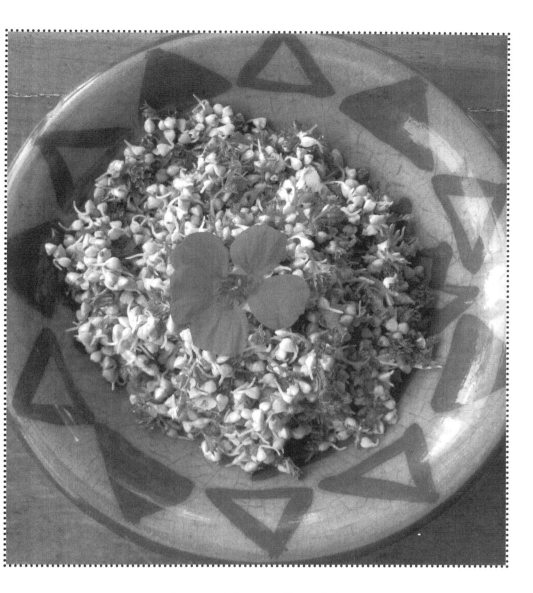

Sprouted Quinoa Tabouleh

Nori Rolls

These are the Japanese seaweed rolls you can buy in sushi bars and most supermarkets. They are easy to make once you have sourced some of the purplish untoasted nori sea vegetable squares.

Lay a square down on a board and arrange a roll of assorted fillings along one side.

Roll the fillings up as in a carpet, and seal the end edge with a little water. Cut across into rolls with a serrated knife. If they come out neatly, you can serve them end-up so you can see the fillings.

You can also cut each nori sheet into four triangles and make filled cones, sealing them with a little water to keep the shape.

Nori rolls are wonderful for raw food because you can be so imaginative with the fillings. Try using whatever left over patés and spreads you have, or work from your memories of vegetarian nori rolls. Sunflower greens, snow pea greens and buckwheat lettuce fit in the rolls very nicely.

If you have some cooked grains you could add some to the fillings, or use grated courgette, sprouted quinoa or buckwheat, or thin strips of young coconut meat as the 'rice'.

Serve them with wasabi, the fiery Japanese horseradish sauce and/or with the **Sweet Ginger Relish** in the **Good Patés, Spreads and Side Dishes** section.

Miso and Almond Butter Nori Rolls
(Protein rich)

These are a little unusual and quite substantial. The quantities make four rolls.

2 tablespoons almond butter
2-3 teaspoons unpasteurised miso
½ teaspoon dried ginger powder
Optional: 1 teaspoon honey or a tiny spoon of pure stevia extract
A pinch of cayenne pepper
A mixture of sprouts and finely chopped salad greens
4 nori sheets

Mix up everything except the nori sheets and the salad greens. Spread the mixture thinly and evenly over the nori sheets. Fill up with sprouts and salad and roll up, using a little water along the inside top edge to seal the rolls. Cut across into short rolls with a sharp serrated knife.

Family Meal Nori

For a meal at home, especially when people have different tastes, set out nori seaweed sheets and a variety of fillings and let people assemble their own. The assembly line is an enjoyable activity, even if it gets messy. Allow for at least three sheets of nori each, and provide a big bowl of salad alongside.

Put out some of these fillings and condiments:

Avocado slices

Thin strips of carrot

Grated courgette 'rice'

Prepared wasabi paste (strong Japanese horseradish sauce. You can buy organic wasabi in tubes in the UK)

Thin asparagus spears wilted in the dehydrator

Thin cucumber strips

Thin tempeh strips (Protein rich), dehydrated if you wish, (see **Tempeh Pieces with Garlic**, perhaps leaving out the garlic for Japanese authenticity)

snow pea greens and sunflower greens

Sprouts

Sweet Ginger Relish

Radish Relish

Tamari

Tastied Sesame Seeds

Soaked sesame seeds

Very finely chopped celery

Finely sliced red sweet pepper or red capsicum

Marinated Shitake Mushrooms

Browned Onions

Interesting leftovers

Everyone puts a sheet of nori on their plates and piles up a 'log' of their selected fillings along one side of the sheet of seaweed. They roll the seaweed around the filling and then, depending on how formal you want to be, either pick them up and eat them, or cut them across into short rolls, and pick those up and eat them.

Mushroom and Courgette Quiche
(Protein rich)

This dish deserves to be called a quiche because it has a pastry crust and is filled with softened vegetables in a savoury custard. The poppy seeds in the crust give it a pleasant crunch. The filling is not that far off a traditional quiche because it is soft and creamy.

This is more involved than many of my recipes, and I would make it for a special occasion.

Pastry crust

2 cups Brazil nuts	Optional: a pinch of sea salt
¼ cup poppy seeds	1 teaspoon of filtered water

Soak the poppy seeds all day or overnight. Rinse, drain and dry them out completely in the dehydrator or in a warm spot on tea towels. I do not soak the Brazil nuts because they need to be completely dry.

Grind the Brazil nuts and optional salt in a food processor until they are sandy or starting to stick together round the sides. Put the ground nuts into a bowl and add the poppy seeds.

Knead and push dough together, adding up to a teaspoonful of water, but certainly not more (that is unless you like very soggy pastry).

Knead the dough until it will just about hold together in lumps, and press it into a pie dish approximately 20cm/8in across, pressing it over the base and up the sides, Neaten the top edge that will show above the filling.

Refrigerate until the filling is ready.

Filling

2 cups finely sliced shitake or Portobello mushrooms
2 cups finely sliced courgettes
1 cup finely sliced mild onions
1 tablespoon of cold pressed olive oil
Optional: ¼ teaspoon herb salt, or a splash of tamari and small
  amount of dried mixed herbs rubbed to powder between your
  fingers, or just the rubbed herbs.

Put the finely sliced vegetables in a large bowl and massage in the cold
pressed olive oil and optional herb salt or tamari and powdered herbs.
Make sure the oil and salt or tamari are mixed in well and that all the
slices are separated. Dehydrate for 1½ hours until softened and tasting
really good.

Savoury custard

10 soaked macadamia nuts	¼ cup filtered water
A tiny piece of garlic	1 teaspoon lemon juice
A few sprigs each of finely chopped fresh basil and oregano	¼ an avocado
	3 teaspoons of ground chia seeds/Mila
A pinch of tumeric	Optional: a splash of tamari
A pinch of black Himalayan sea salt (for the egg taste)	

Blend together the macadamia nuts, garlic, lemon juice, turmeric, salt
and water to get as smooth a custard as you can. Add the chia/Mila and
keep blending. Lastly add the avocado and blend again until it has mixed
in completely.

Reserving a few vegetable pieces for a garnish, mix the vegetables into
the custard and smooth into the pastry shell. Garnish with the reserved
vegetables and serve or refrigerate. It is better at room temperature than
cold from the fridge.

Indonesian Satay Sticks
(Protein rich)

Serve little satay sticks, or larger kebab sticks, laden with pieces of marinated and lightly dehydrated tempeh, mushrooms, sweet red pepper pieces , small mild onion quarters and courgettes along with **Indonesian Satay Sauce** and you have a rich and delicious satay. See the photo on page 121. It would be good with a light salad of shredded lettuce, Chinese bean sprouts and other sprouts.

Depending on the size of the sticks you can find and whether you want delicate little satays or larger main dish satay/kebabs, cut suitably-sized chunks of marinated tempeh and/or vegetables and thread them on to the sticks. Paint them with sesame oil on a pastry brush and dehydrate for an hour or more until they are warmed through and have an interesting chewy surface texture. For saltier satays you could mix a little tamari with the sesame oil, but remember that the satay sauce is salty. If the sauce is too thick for easy dipping, dilute it with a little coconut water or filtered water.

Japanese Misodare Vegetables
(Protein rich)

This dish is a thin warm soupy sauce over finely sliced oriental vegetables. I modelled this on what I had in a Japanese café, which was very hot, over-garlicky, very sweet, and deliciously complex. All the flavours were pulled together by the miso. This version is less sweet, but you could add more maple syrup, yacon syrup, honey, agave or pure stevia extract to taste. It is good as it is, with the soupy sauce, or, you can make noodles with 2 or 3 courgettes with a julienne cutter or *Benriner*, or similar and stir them into the sauce too. Serves 4

1 cup shitake mushrooms
4 cups Chinese bean sprouts
4 cups Chinese cabbage or ordinary white cabbage, finely sliced
4-5 large cloves of garlic, finely grated or crushed
½ cup spring onions/scallions finely sliced lengthwise
2 tablespoons aged miso
Optional: 1 tablespoon tamari
1 tablespoon yacon syrup, maple syrup or a little pure stevia extract to taste.
¼ teaspoon cayenne pepper
2-3 tablespoons **Tastied Sesame Seeds** or soaked sesame seeds.
1 tablespoon cold pressed sesame oil
1 small carrot
Optional: 3 courgettes for making fresh raw noodles
1 cup filtered water

Slice the mushrooms finely, reserving the stalks for something else. Mix the oil and half the miso together with the crushed garlic, cayenne pepper and yacon syrup/maple syrup/stevia to a thin cream and mix into the bean sprouts, mushrooms, spring onions and Chinese cabbage. Leave to marinate or spread the mixture out on a silicone sheet on a dehydrator tray and dehydrate for a couple of hours to wilt the vegetables.

If you wish, turn the courgettes into noodles, as in the **Good Equipment** section. Mix the rest of the miso into a thin broth with the cup of water, and when ready to serve, add the vegetables.

Adjust the seasonings, adding a little more water if it is too salty or the tamari if it is not salty enough. Add the noodles at this point if you wish, being careful not to break them. If you add noodles you might want to drizzle in another tablespoon of sesame oil. Stir over a very low heat with your clean finger until comfortably warm. Garnish with plenty of **Tastied Sesame Seeds** or soaked sesame seeds, very lightly ground in a grinder or pulsed in a blender.

Variation: Crush or finely grate a small piece of ginger and add to the vegetables before marinating them.

....

Oriental Raw Stir
(Protein rich)

This recipe is for a raw meal to have instead of a Chinese takeaway. It tastes rich without actually being very greasy. It is a recipe you can play with. Add some greens in the form of thin purple sprouting broccoli. Add sliced shitake mushrooms. Spice things up with ginger or cayenne. You do not have to be too precise with quantities and you can adjust the seasonings to suit your taste.

3 Cups finely sliced cabbage

I cup soaked, chopped macadamia nuts or pine nuts

I bag fresh Chinese bean sprouts, approximately 8 cups

I grated carrot

2-3 courgettes, either grated coarsely or cut into thickish julienne strips

3 tablespoons cold pressed sesame oil

A very small piece of garlic

I dessert spoon lemon juice

Optional: I tablespoon agave syrup or honey, or a tiny spoon or drop of pure stevia extract

Optional: A splash of tamari

2 finely sliced spring onions

Make the noodles by peeling away the whole courgette lengthwise with a julienne cutter or with a *Benriner* or similar, or just use a coarse grater and make 'rice'.

Crush the garlic. Prepare the all vegetables and stir together with the seasonings, being careful not to break the noodles.

Leave for several hours for the flavours to mix in and for the vegetables to wilt for a more 'cooked' texture. You can dehydrate the stir-raw for an hour to warm it through and wilt it further.

Five Spice Raw Stir
(Protein rich)

Make the **Oriental Raw Stir** once as above, for the experience, and then make it in the same way but add a level teaspoon of Chinese five spice powder.

Creating Raw Stirs

Once you have made and eaten a couple of 'raw stirs', you will see the potential for creating an infinite variety. Make them more spicy with cayenne pepper. Add chopped herbs such as coriander and basil.

Add finely sliced red sweet peppers. Use finely sliced Chinese cabbage or red cabbage instead of white cabbage. Try different vegetable combinations.

Add thinly-sliced shitake mushrooms or fresh raw sweet corn scraped from the cob. Experiment with more and less oil, garlic, sweetness and spiciness.

By adding warm filtered water and perhaps a little miso, you can turn the raw stir into a noodle broth. However you develop your own creations, marinate the ingredients together for several hours before serving because that is what changes the texture to something more like a regular stir fry.

If you are making a noodle broth with vegetables, marinate everything first before adding the warm water and miso.

• •

Chinese Five-Spice Seaweed Noodles

This recipe is for the ultimate in raw comfort food. The noodles are raw and processed from seaweed. You can buy them online, at a price. See the **Good Resources** section. Once in a while they are definitely worth it. Stretch the packet to two people, if you feel kind. Serve with a salad of oriental vegetables such as Chinese cabbage, Chinese bean sprouts, finely sliced greens and finely sliced spring onions.

1 packet of seaweed noodles
1 level teaspoon of Chinese five-spice powder
Optional: tamari to taste
A small piece of ginger
A small piece of garlic
1 tablespoon lemon juice
2-4 tablespoons cold pressed sesame oil
Optional: 1 teaspoon of honey or a tiny spoon or drop of pure stevia
  extract

Open the packet and soak the seaweed noodles in filtered water for an hour. Blend 2 tablespoons of the oil and the other sauce ingredients together. Rinse and drain the noodles. Stir in the sauce, adding more oil if you wish, and enjoy.

This recipe also works very well with courgette noodles. Start with noodles made from two courgettes, and add more if the sauce will spread that far.

Cucumber Sandwiches
(Protein rich)

These can be pretty little canapés or lunch box staples. Simply cut cucumber slices and sandwich them together with a paté. If you cut the cucumber slices on the diagonal the sandwiches will be a little bigger.

Pecan Cream Risotto
(Protein rich)

The rice for this dish is grated parsnips. You can also use grated courgettes. I have also made it with a mixture of sweet corn scraped from the cob with sprouted lentils. The parsnips or courgettes are a little more like risotto. It is concentrated and rich, so not for huge portions. Serves 4

Cream

½ cup pecans, soaked for a day or night and rinsed
2 tablespoons cold pressed olive oil
4 teaspoons lemon juice
A few fresh basil and oregano leaves
Optional: a pinch of sea salt
Filtered water as needed

Blend well, adding a little water if necessary.

Rice

1 cup grated parsnip or courgette

Stir the 'rice' into the cream. Parsnips can soak up water so add more if it is too dry. Garnish with a few finely chopped onions.

Lasagne

The special equipment you need for this is a potato peeler. The pasta layers are thin ribbons of courgette made by skinning down the side of the courgette until nothing much is left. Use the remainders for something else, perhaps chopping it finely into a mixed salad.

The sauce layers are pesto, red capsicum pepper sauce and avocado sauce. You could make the lasagne with just the pesto or tomato sauce plus the avocado sauce, in which case double up that sauce. You could add a layer of very thinly sliced vine-ripened tomatoes. Serves 3-4 people.

4-5 courgettes Extra cold pressed olive oil	**Pesto** – choose from the pesto recipes

Red Pepper Sauce

A large red capsicum pepper or a couple of sweet red pointed peppers. ¼ small red onion 1 small garlic clove	A shake of tamari I tablespoon cold pressed olive oil Juice of ¼ lemon

Blend all together and adjust lemon and tamari to taste. It is similar to a tomato sauce but without the acidity of tomatoes.

Avocado Sauce

This bears some very slight resemblance to a cheese sauce because it contributes creaminess.

1 ripe avocado A pinch of sea salt or a splash of tamari	A squeeze of lemon juice A tablespoon of cold pressed olive oil

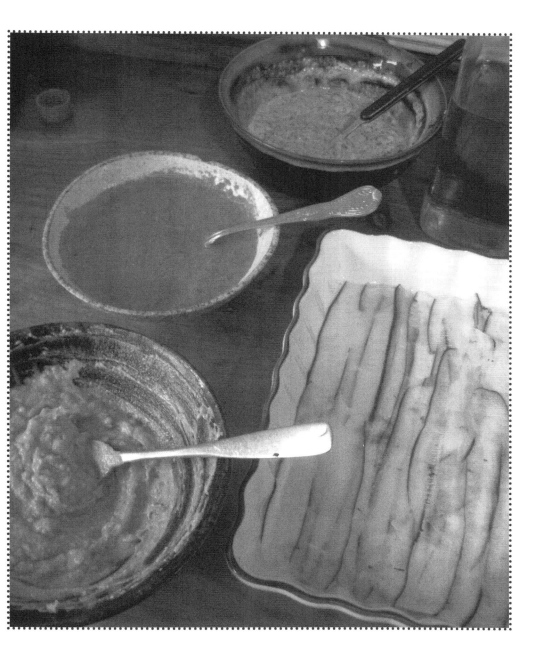

Assembling Lasagne

Mash all together till smooth, adding more salt or tamari and lemon to taste. To assemble the lasagne, drizzle a little olive oil into an oblong serving dish and smooth it over the base. Add a layer of overlapping courgette ribbons. Alternate layers of sauce and courgette until you have used everything up, finishing with the avocado sauce. Garnish with thin slices of red sweet pepper or capsicum, sliced olives and/or **Sunflower Pecorino Shards** sprinkled over at the last moment.

....

Pizzas

Are these pizzas? Do raw creations need to be like their cooked counterparts? These creations certainly look like pizzas and they are brilliant table centrepieces. They have crunchy or chewy bases. They are large, round and colourful with interesting toppings and textures, and they can be eaten in slices. What I know is that I like them. I have served them to people, some new to raw foods, who have enjoyed them so much that they were not comparing them at all, just enjoying them, intrigued.

These two versions are a carbohydrate rich pizza with a buckwheat base, and a protein rich pizza with a sunflower and flax seed base. If you do not have a dehydrator, make a protein rich base with the **Courgette and Mushroom Quiche** pastry recipe. The carbohydrate rich pizza has an avocado 'cheese' topping and a crunchy base, while the protein rich pizza has a macadamia nut 'cheese' and a chewy base. Both have sweet red pepper or red capsicum sauces which taste wonderful and avoid the acidity of tomatoes.

The recipes may look complicated but, like the lasagne recipe, when you have made them once they are straightforward, no more complicated than traditional cooked pizzas.

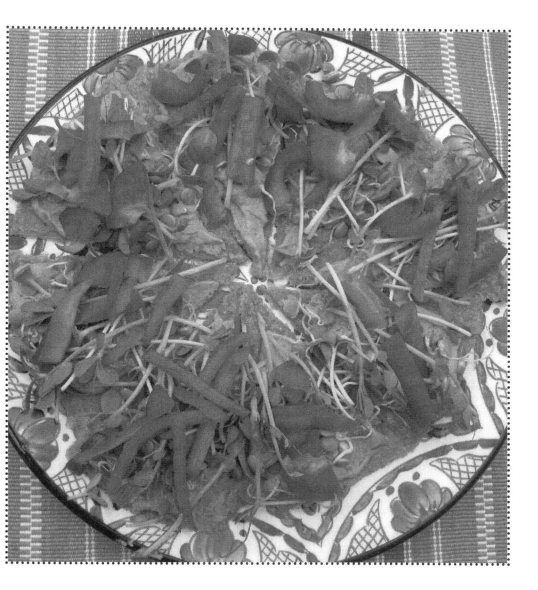

Pizza

Pizza Toppings

Make your choice from:

- **Marinated Shitake Mushrooms**
- **Browned Onions**
- **Garlic Tempeh Pieces** (Protein rich)
- Thinly sliced red capsicum or sweet red pepper
- Sliced olives
- **Sunflower Pecorino Shreds** (Protein rich)
- Capers
- **Aubergine or Courgette Rashers,** cut in pieces
- Chopped fresh herbs
- Drizzled cold pressed olive oil
- Sprouts and tray greens – as ever!
- Thin asparagus spears, brushed with oil and wilted in a dehydrator

••

Avocado and Sweet Red Pepper Pizza
(Carbohydrate rich)

Make a pizza base from the **Crunchy Base for Pizza and Quiche** recipe in the **Good Dehydrated Creations** section. Make the **Red Pepper Sauce** from the **Lasagne** recipe and thicken it a little by blending in an inch or so of peeled courgette. Make the **Avocado Sauce** from the **Lasagne** recipe. At the last minute before serving, spread the base with the **Red Pepper Sauce** and then the **Avocado Sauce,** and add toppings of your choice.

Makes one large pizza.

Macadamia Nut and Basil Cheese and Sweet Red Pepper Pizza (Protein rich)

Makes one large pizza.

Make a **Sunflower and Flax Seed Pizza Base** from the end of the **Good Dehydrated Creations** section. Make the **Red Pepper Sauce** from the **Lasagne** recipe and thicken it with 2-3 teaspoons of ground chia seeds or Mila. Make the **Macadamia and Carrot Cheesy Sauce** from the **Good Sauces** section, blending in a few sprigs of fresh basil.

At the last moment spread the red pepper sauce and then the cheesy sauce on the base, letting some of the red pepper sauce show through. Add toppings of your choice and serve with salads and sprouts, probably to appreciative silent applause.

Good
Dehydrated Creations

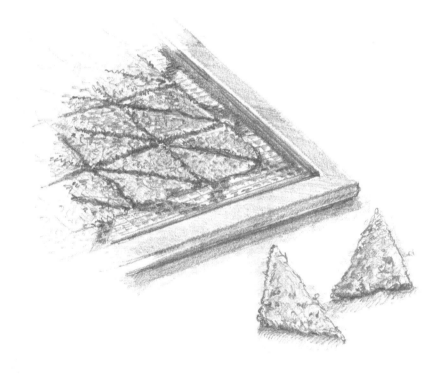

Corn Chips still warm from the dehydrator

Pretty much everything dried out in a dehydrator, savoury or sweet, is gathered in this section. That way you can ignore it all if you do not have one, or investigate all the possibilities if you do. Tip: try the **Gingernut Cookies** first.

The point of the dehydrator is to change and develop tastes and textures without overheating the food. That way the enzymes are retained for better digestion. Some nutrition may be lost through oxidation in the dehydration process, but far less than is destroyed by the heat of cooking.

Keep your dehydrator at around 115°F/46°C to dry out crackers and other raw creations. Much lower and they would take too long. You can go a little higher when you want to heat a thicker moist dish. That is because the moisture and lack of heat in the food is working against the heat circulating in the dehydrator, and as a result the food will not get overheated, unless you forget it for ages!

I love the variety of dishes that dehydrating brings to raw eating, and make all sorts of dried food for travelling and for variety at home.

Something very good about dehydrated crackers, crisps and sprinkles is that they keep so well. The completely crisped foods keep for days, or longer, in air tight containers, unless, as often happens, they get discovered and eaten.

I have been artfully vague with the length of drying times, partly because so much depends on the humidity and air temperature of your kitchen. Besides, it is good to be around when your creations are drying so that you can whip them out when they are ready. Or you can work with the timer. Or you can go off whistling or go to sleep, happy knowing that nothing will burn or be spoiled if you do leave it in too long.

Dehydrated crackers are becoming more popular and many good health food shops now stock them. Buying an occasional packet might give you new ideas. The first few recipes are for a variety of crackers, and then there are recipes for all kinds of tasty creations. I tend to have a day every week or two when I make various things at once, using most or all of the dehydrator trays. That saves time, electricity and effort.

Flax, Almond, Onion and Ginger Crackers
(Protein rich)

These are good all-purpose crackers to eat as snacks or with spreads

1 cup flax seeds
½ cup almonds, soaked for a day or night
½ medium white onion
A Brazil nut-sized chunk of ginger
2 tablespoons of cold pressed olive oil
optional: 1 tablespoon tamari
1 cup filtered filtered water + extra

Soak the almonds the morning or evening before.

Leave the flax to soak in the cup of water while processing the almonds, onion, ginger, oil and tamari with the minimum of water to mix to quite a smooth paste.

Stir the paste into the soaked flax and leave the mixture to sit for half an hour for the flavours to mix.

Spread thinly on non-stick drying sheets on the mesh dehydrator trays and score into squares or rectangles. Dehydrate for a day or a night. To speed up drying a little, when the mixture is dry enough to do so, flip each sheet over onto another tray and peel the paper off. Then continue drying until the crackers are completely crisp.

Carrot and Coriander Crackers

The carrot and coriander combination is just as good in crackers as it is in soups, perhaps because they are both quite sweet tastes.

1½ cups of flax seed/linseed
At least a cup of chopped coriander
1 very large carrot or equivalent in smaller carrots
1 small red onion
Optional: 1 tablespoon tamari
Optional: 1 large pinch sea salt
2 tablespoons cold pressed olive oil
1 cup pumpkin seeds (measured before soaking) soaked
1½ cups filtered water

Process everything together till grainy but not completely smooth.

Stir into the flax in a large bowl and leave to thicken and soften the flax. Stir again and spread thinly onto non-stick drying sheets. Score into squares or oblongs. Dehydrate for several hours until you can flip each sheet over onto another tray and peel off the backing sheet. Then dehydrate all day or overnight until completely crisp.

··

Seaweed and Walnut Crackers

These are another example of the infinite variety of crackers in the raw food universe, thank heavens.

1 ½ cups flax seeds/linseed
1 cup of walnuts that have been soaked, rinsed and dehydrated (or
  just soaked and rinsed, in which case use slightly less water) and
  processed into very tiny pieces
Optional: 1-3 tablespoons of tamari
2 handfuls of soft seaweed such as dulse
½ a clove of garlic, finely crushed, or a pinch of garlic powder
3 cups filtered water

Mix the water and one cup of the flax seeds in a powerful blender with the seaweed, tamari and garlic. Tip the mixture into a bowl with the walnuts and the rest of the flax and stir well. Spread out onto non-stick drying sheets ¼-⅓ in/ ½ cm thick. Score it in cracker-size squares and dehydrate till firm enough to flip and peel off the non-stick drying sheet. Dehydrate overnight or all day until completely crisp.

Broccoli Crackers

These came from a self-imposed challenge. I was not sure how the strong taste of broccoli would be in a cracker, but I had a small head of broccoli to use up before going away. I made crackers for the journey and really like them. They are quite highly spiced to balance the broccoli. Process everything except the flax and Mila/chia seeds and the water.

1 small head broccoli
2 tablespoons cold pressed olive
  oil
½ a small red onion
1 teaspoon cumin seeds
1 large pinch cayenne
1 teaspoon turmeric
2 tablespoons Mila/chia seeds

2 tablespoons flax seeds/linseed
Optional: 2 tablespoons tamari
1 level teaspoon of powdered
  ginger or 2 teaspoons of finely-
  grated fresh ginger
½ a small lemon
6 tablespoons filtered water

Then add in those and process a little longer to mix well. Spread ¼ inch/ ½ centimetre thick on non-stick drying sheets on dehydrator trays and dehydrate all day or overnight. As always with crackers, you can flip them over onto another tray after a couple of hours and peel off the drying sheet to speed up the drying time.

I wonder, how would these be if made with cauliflower?

· ·

Japanese Seaweed and Flax Crackers

2 cups light or dark flax seeds/linseed
3 cups filtered water
1 packed cup 'sea salad' or other light thin seaweed such as dulse or nori

Soak the flax in the water for at least an hour until it is a thick porridge.

Cut up any long strands of seaweed and stir it into the flax. Stir well and spread thinly on non-stick drying sheets.

Dehydrate until dry enough to remove the drying sheets. Continue drying until crisp, about 6 hours. Break into uneven pieces.

You can vary this recipe by mixing in a little honey or a tiny spoon or drop of pure stevia extract, and/or a crushed garlic clove.

For a saltier cracker, perhaps to break up into smaller pieces and use as a sprinkle, add a tablespoon of tamari.

Tamari-glazed Sunflower Twigs

These were a lucky invention from a batch of sunflower crackers that came out wrong. When they were dehydrated and I had decided I did not like them, I mixed up a solution of a little cayenne in tamari and painted each one very lightly with the solution on a pastry brush, and then dried them further.

They are very tasty without being too salty. The taste is a little like that salty yeast spread taste that they say you either hate or love.
Process the sunflower seeds, garlic, carrot, onion and lemon juice together until quite smooth.

2 cups of sunflower seeds soaked for several hours or overnight	¼ cup each flax/linseed and Mila/chia seeds
1 small piece of garlic	Filtered water as necessary
1 small carrot	1 tablespoon of tamari
¼ small mild onion	A pinch of cayenne pepper
1 tablespoon lemon juice	

Grind the chia/Mila and flax separately and add to the mixture. Process to mix well, adding water little by little if necessary for a thick dough.

Spread the mixture thinly over non-stick drying sheets on three dehydrator trays and score into long thin twig strips. If you have a zig-zag edged pastry cutter, use that to make rough-edged twigs. Dehydrate for most of the day until crisp.

Mix the cayenne into the tamari in a small cup. Using a pastry brush, paint along each twig with the tamari. There should be just enough for the three trays. Dehydrate for another half an hour to dry the glaze. Then, have a party or take them to a party and share. They will vanish. Everyone will love you.

Corn Chips

If you know that tomorrow evening you want to snuggle up watching a screen and eating corn chips and dip, make these tonight and make the dip tomorrow. It makes a bowlful that will soon empty.

Make sure that the corn you use is GMO free. Apparently in the States that is quite an issue because of pollen drift. Only use organic corn and, especially if making these regularly, do your homework to make sure the corn is from a safe source.

You can vary this by adding a chopped sweet red repper or red capsicum to the food processor, as well or instead of the herbs.

4 cups fresh raw corn kernels scraped from the cobs, or fresh frozen raw corn thawed to room temperature.	¼ teaspoon cayenne pepper
	½ cup flax seeds/linseed, ground
	2 tablespoons tamari
	2 tablespoons filtered water
½ bunch of coriander leaves and stalks (or parsley, or basil, or a mixture)	3 tablespoons cold pressed olive oil
	1 cup sprouted and dried buckwheat

In a food processor, process the herbs and corn to a mush, but still with some texture. Add the cayenne, flax seeds, tamari, water and oil and process enough to mix everything well.

Turn the mixture into a large bowl and add the buckwheat. Stir it in and spread the mixture thinly over non-stick drying sheets on dehydrator trays. Score into large triangles.

Dehydrate for an hour or two until the mixture is firm enough to flip the sheets over and peel back the drying sheet. Then dehydrate all day or overnight until completely crisp.

I particularly like these with the buckwheat in them, and they dry more quickly, but you can add another cup of corn instead of the buckwheat and proceed in the same way, allowing a longer drying time.

Corn Tortillas

With the extra corn and not the buckwheat, the mixture makes good semi-soft corn tortillas. These are the tortillas you can see in the tacos on the front cover. Spread the mixture in corn tortilla-size circles and dehydrate until they are firm and still pliable. Double the recipe to serve 4.

Then, fill with any, or all, of these: sprouts, **Red Pepper Salsa, Guacamole, Tempeh Mince,** salad, **Sunflower Sour Cream, Mild Pepper Sauce** (with extra cayenne for hot pepper sauce), finely chopped coriander leaves and **Sunflower Pecorino Shards**. People I know like to see all the fillings on the table and to compose their own masterpieces.

....

Japanese Kale Crisps

Who would have thought this dark leafy vegetable that strikes terror into the hearts of some who lived through school dinners could be turned into something delicious and crunchy, and worth taking to eat in movies?

4 cups of very tightly packed chopped kale, minus the stems
1 tablespoon cold pressed olive or sesame oil
1 tablespoon tamari
1 tablespoon honey/agave/yacon, or none, or a tiny spoon or drop of
  pure stevia extract
1 teaspoon crushed fresh ginger
¼ teaspoon crushed fresh garlic

Tear up the kale and reserve the biggest stalks for juicing. Measure the other ingredients and massage them into the kale in a large bowl. Spread on mesh dehydrator sheets with spaces between for several hours until completely crisp.

Oatcakes

Oats are warming, and if you live in a cold climate warming foods are very good! These oatcakes are delicious 'buttered' with ripe avocado or raw buttery spreads. Because dehydrators are on the slow side it is good to make them very thin, so I cut them in quite big squares. They do roll up at the edges and do not look very tidy, but who cares if they are there in the tin when you come home cold and hungry.

The point is to use raw oats and most on sale are not. I buy mine online. See **Good Resources**.

2 cups raw oats, whole if possible, or rolled but not steamed.
½ cup chia seeds
Optional: 1 teaspoon of sea salt
1½ cups filtered water + 1 further cup
Soak the oats overnight or all day. If whole, leave them to sprout for a
  further day and night, rinsing each day.

Soak the chia seeds in 1½ cups water and leave to absorb it all. Blend the oats and sea salt with 1 cup of water, leaving the mixture slightly coarse if you like rough oatcakes. Stir into the chia seeds in a bowl and stir well.

Spread ⅜ inch / ¾ centimetre thick on non-stick drying sheets and make into quite large squares.

Dehydrate until dried enough to flip over onto the mesh sheets and peel back the non-stick sheets. Dehydrate 12+ hours until completely dry.

Store in an airtight container.

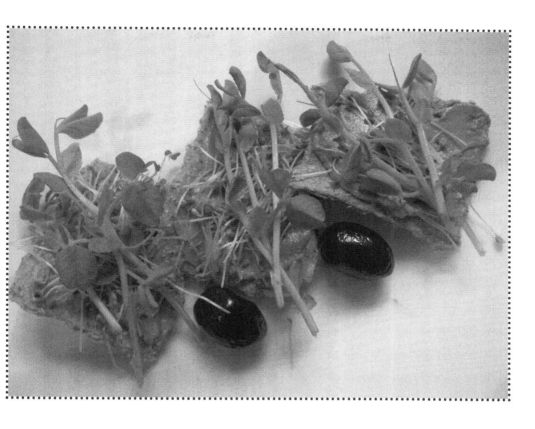

Oatcakes with Guacamole, snow pea greens,
sunflower greens and olives

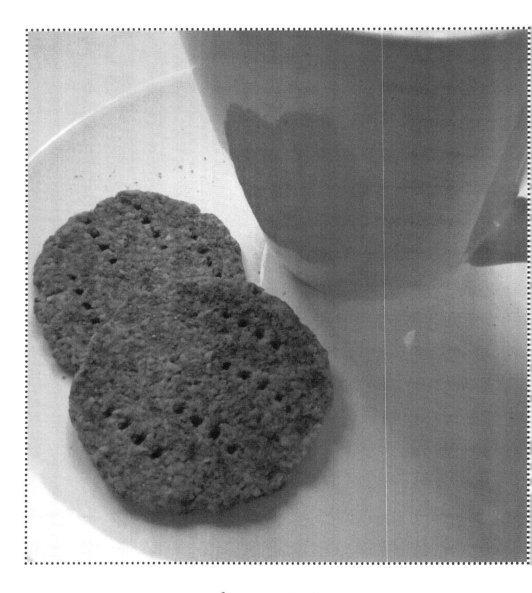

Gingernut Cookies

Gingernut Cookies

These are my favourites because they are sweet, crunchy and gingery and just as nice as the original baked version, or nicer. You can even dunk them in hot drinks. The sweetness is from the carrot juice and from pure stevia extract, and the ginger overpowers any hint of stevia after-taste so that even people who often do not like stevia in some things like these, a lot. They are brilliant low-sugar sweet biscuits. The salt makes the authentic traditional taste but you do not need it.

2 cups Brazil nuts, soaked overnight
1 cup carrot juice
1 cup ginger juice
½ cup Mila/ground chia seeds
½ cup carrot fibre from making the carrot juice
Optional: ½ teaspoon sea salt
¼ teaspoon pure stevia powder or a few drops of pure stevia liquid
    extract to taste.

In a food processor, process the nuts and carrot juice for a couple of minutes or less. The mixture should still retain the graininess of the little particles of Brazil nuts. Turn the mixture into a bowl and knead in the other ingredients by hand. Roll into balls and flatten into circles about ⅓ cm / ¼ inch thick on non-stick drying sheets. Mark with a fork to decorate. Dehydrate for a couple of hours until firm enough to flip and peel back the drying sheet. Dehydrate overnight or all day until completely crisp. If people did not eat them up so quickly they would probably keep well.

Cheesy Kale Crisps
(Protein rich)

These are quite substantial with the sunflowers and are good as part of a meal or in packed lunches. I am told that these do taste cheesy. They keep well, if you can forget that they are there.

1 cup sunflower seeds, soaked over night or all day, rinsed and
  drained
1 tablespoon lemon juice
1 teaspoon of paprika pepper
1/8th teaspoon cayenne pepper
1 small clove of garlic (crushed unless you have a powerful blender)
2 tablespoons olive oil
1-2 tablespoons tamari
¼ cup filtered water, more if necessary
¼ teaspoon turmeric
3 cups of very tightly packed kale with the stalks removed and torn to
  pieces (save the stalks for your green juice)

Prepare the kale by rinsing it and drying it between tea towels, cutting out the stems and tearing the leaves into crisp-size pieces. Blend all the other ingredients, using the minimum amount of water for a thick smooth cream. Massage the cream into the kale pieces and spread them out on mesh dehydrator trays. Dehydrate for several hours until bone dry.

Crisp Pollen and Sesame Bars

These are low sugar snack bars sweetened with stevia and, if you wish, flavoured with a little honey. They contain bee pollen because it is such a nourishing food, and because it adds its own sweetness. If you want even less sugar you can leave the honey out and add a little vanilla instead.

1 cup soaked sesame seeds, soaked for a few hours or starting to sprout if possible. How long it will take to sprout them depends on the quality of the seeds. Use them after 36 hours whether or not they show signs of sprouting.
1 cup Mila/chia seeds
Optional: 1 tablespoon honey
Optional: 1 teaspoon vanilla essence
A heaped tiny spoon or two drops of pure stevia extract, or more to taste
½ cup filtered water + 2 tablespoons
½ cup of pollen

Mix everything together except the stevia. Leave for half an hour to soften the pollen and to let the chia/Mila soak up the water. Add a little stevia to taste and mix well again.

Spread onto a non-stick drying sheet and pat out into a large square about ½ cm/ ⅓ in thick.

Mark into bar shapes.

Dehydrate for an hour or two until you can flip the bars and pull back the drying sheet.

Dehydrate for the rest of the day or overnight until completely crisp.

Brazil Nut Burgers

Put these in round cabbage leaf 'buns' along with **Red Pepper Ketchup** and assorted sprouts for delicious and surprisingly filling burgers.

2 celery stalks
1 medium – large carrot
A handful of dulse
1 medium courgette
2 small – medium mild onions
1 teaspoon each of dried sage and oregano or marjoram, or 2
  teaspoons each of fresh, finely chopped
1 cup Brazil nuts
2 tablespoons tamari
2 tablespoons lemon juice
¼ cup of ground chia/Mila
¼ cup of flax seeds/linseed

Process everything except the chia/Mila and the flax in a food processor. Turn the mixture into a bowl and stir in the chia/Mila and the flax seeds. Form into thin burger shapes, adding a little water if necessary and put them close together on non-stick drying sheets. Dehydrate for a few hours until drying on the outside and moist, not soggy, on the inside.

You could add a little more water to some of the mixture and spread it out thinly on a non-stick drying sheet, score the mixture into squares and make some crackers.

Sweet Potato Wrapped Chipolatas

These look intriguing and the sweet potato wrap makes an interesting texture. You can make the same mixture into plain chipolatas, patties and burgers.

They taste good with radish and ginger relish or as part of a 'full British' breakfast.

2 carrots, grated finely
2 courgettes, grated finely
½ a very finely chopped red or white onion
A pinch each of cayenne powder and garlic powder or finely-crushed fresh garlic
1 cup of walnuts that have been soaked well, rinsed, dehydrated and processed to a grainy texture, a step before they threaten to turn into walnut butter
¼ cup ground flax seed/linseed
I teaspoon mixed dried herbs or a tablespoon of very finely chopped fresh herbs
I tablespoon unpasteurised sweet miso
I tablespoon tamari
I squeeze lemon juice

Knead all together with your hands and leave to thicken slightly.

Wrapping (optional): Shave long slices from a sweet potato with a potato peeler and cut them in half lengthwise. Place in the dehydrator for half an hour so they wilt and become pliable.

Form the chipolata mixture into thin little sausage shapes and roll a wilted sweet potato slice round each in a spiral along the length of the shape, letting the chipolata mixture show through. It does not matter if things get sticky; just keep going. Dehydrate for several hours until gently crisped on the outside.

Serve sprinkled with sesame seeds and with beautiful pink **Radish Relish**.

Tempeh and Onion Mince
(Protein rich)

This is a good savoury mixture for wraps and tortillas, and to put on raw pizzas. Or sprinkle over red pepper sauce on courgette pasta. Then you could sprinkle **Sunflower Pecorino** on the top for a complex Italian pasta treat.

½ teaspoon each dried sage and dried thyme	1 small-medium clove of garlic, crushed
A 220gm/8oz block of fresh tempeh	2 tablespoons cold pressed olive oil
2 medium mild onions	1½ tablespoons tamari

Cut or crumble the tempeh into little pieces and put them in a bowl. Add the finely chopped onions, crushed garlic, olive oil and the tamari and mix well with your hands. Spread the mixture out on a non-stick drying sheet and dehydrate for several hours until the onions have softened slightly, the tempeh has taken up the oil and tamari, and everything has started to dry slightly.

....

Tempeh Pieces with Garlic
(Protein rich)

1 8oz/225gm block tempeh	1 tablespoon cold pressed olive oil
1 crushed clove of garlic	1 tablespoon tamari

Mix the garlic, tamari and oil together and allow to marinate in a bowl while cutting or crumbling the tempeh into little pieces. Mix all together with your hands.

Spread on a dehydrator tray with a non-stick drying sheet and dehydrate for a couple of hours until the pieces are warm and have dried slightly on the outsides while still soft inside. Serve as a salad or soup sprinkle, over raw pasta or in wraps and tacos.

....

Aubergine or Courgette Rashers

These are delectably rich and chewy and a rasher or two adds something special to a meal. The liquid aminos are particularly good for creating the salty smoky bacon taste, but tamari is fine too. Eat them when they are juicy and soft, or dehydrate them for chewier and crispy textures.

1 aubergine or a couple of courgettes
2 tablespoons liquid aminos
3 tablespoons cold pressed walnut or sesame oil
1 tablespoon filtered water
½ teaspoon honey/yacon syrup or a tiny spoon/1 drop of pure stevia
  extract
1 tablespoon lemon juice

Halve the aubergine/courgettes lengthwise and slice thinly into rashers, tapering the rasher cuts for 'bacon' that is crispier at one end. Mix the marinade ingredients in a wide bowl and layer in the rashers.

Marinate all day or night, spooning the juice around occasionally if you are awake. If you wish, you can then dehydrate them for crispier bacon.

Stuffing Balls
(Carbohydrate rich)

These are a tasty accompaniment for a traditional meal. You could make tiny ones and stuff them in tortillas as you might falafels, with sprouts, salad and a sauce.

2 level teaspoons of dried or 1 tablespoon finely chopped fresh sage
2 level teaspoons dried or 1 tablespoon finely chopped fresh thyme
2 small mild onions
2 tablespoons cold pressed olive oil
½ cup of dried sprouted buckwheat – see the **Buckwheaties** recipe
Optional: a splash of tamari
2 teaspoons filtered water
2 courgettes
2 tablespoons chia seeds/Mila

Chop the onions very finely and mix with the oil, tamari and water. Spread on a silicone sheet and dehydrate for a couple of hours until softened.

Peel the courgettes, saving the peel to slice finely into a salad or for green juice.

Grind the chia seeds and process them or the Mila with the herbs and the courgettes.

Grind the buckwheat to flour in a grinder or powerful blender that can handle dry ingredients.

Add the buckwheat flour to the courgette mixture and process briefly. Turn the mixture into large bowl and mix in the onions.

Roll into balls about 1½ inch/2 centimetres diameter, or smaller, and dehydrate for a few hours until crispy on the outside and still soft inside.

Sunflower Pecorino Shards
(Protein rich)

These are delicious crispy cheesy pieces to crumble over Italian dishes and salads. Try them on courgette pasta or on a raw pizza.

2 cups sunflower seeds, soaked overnight (and, if time, sprouted for 24 hours)
½ teaspoon sea salt or a splash of tamari
A pinch of cayenne pepper
A minute piece of garlic
½ teaspoon turmeric
The juice of half a lemon
2 tablespoons cold pressed olive oil
Filtered water

Rinse and drain the sunflower seeds. Puree everything in a processor or powerful blender, adding water a spoon at a time, using just sufficient to make a thick smooth cream. The turmeric is for a cheese colour and the cayenne gives it a slight warmth. Spread the cream out as thinly as you can on non-stick drying sheets. Dehydrate till completely crisp, perhaps 4-6 hours, and break into uneven pieces. Store in an airtight container.

Celery 'Salt'

This tastes more salty than you might expect and is good for rounding out the flavour of savoury creations. Slice stalks of celery thinly and cover mesh dehydrator trays with them. Dehydrate until they are completely dry and grind to a powder. They shrink down, so slice up plenty of celery at a time. They take ages to dry and so you might want to fill spare dehydrator trays with them when you are making something else. Keep the powder in an airtight jar and use as a good salty seasoning. Try substituting it for tamari and sea salt.

....

Garlic Powder and Onion Powder

Make powerful onion and garlic powder in the same way as the celery salt. The garlic powder in particular has a very strong taste, so use minute quantities until you get used to it.

....

Sea Vegetable Sprinkle

When you harvest your own sea vegetables (and make sure you learn where and what pick to from someone who knows) or buy bulk seaweed, especially seaweed such as kelp which is quite thick and not that nice either in soft or crispy pieces in raw meals, you can turn it into a very useful seaweed powder to use as a condiment instead of sea salt and tamari in savoury recipes. I use it daily to make sure I get enough sea vegetables, for their iodine as well as protein, minerals and more.

I think you do need a powerful blender to make this, or you could make very small quanties in a grinder. Pull out half the trays in the dehydrator to give more depth over each tray. Fill the trays with pieces of seaweed and dehydrate until they are completely, utterly, dry. Squashing as much as you can into the blender each time, grind the seaweed to powder or to tiny granules, or a mixture (depends on the kind of seaweed and how long you keep blending) Do not lift the lid off the blender until the powder has had a couple of minutes to settle, or you will risk breathing in a lot of seaweed dust! Stored in an airtight jar, it keeps indefinitely.

· ·

Green Crisps
(Protein rich)

I invented these as a palatable and convenient way of taking spirulina, chlorella and bluegreen algae powders when away from home, but now I make them for use at home as well. They have a green taste worth acquiring as they are an extremely nourishing snack for keeping up energy levels. Because they are so energizing they are best eaten before evening, unless you want to stay up late! They are very thin and take less time to dehydrate than crackers. Eat as a snack and sprinkle on meals.

1 medium courgette
1 cup kale or broccoli leaves, minus their stems and packed in tightly
Optional: 1 tablespoon tamari
1½ tablespoons lemon juice
1 tablespoon cold pressed olive oil

¼ cup soaked and dried almonds, or a heaped ¼ cup of soaked
  almonds
A small garlic clove, crushed
I tablespoon each of chlorella, spirulina and blue green algae powders
  (or 3 tablespoons of whichever you have)
¼ cup of chia seeds/Mila

Blend everything together in a food processor, adding a little water if
necessary to make a thick, spreadable cream.

Spread as thinly as possible over silicone sheets on 4 or 5 dehydrator
sheets. Dry for several hours until completely crisp.

A variation on this theme is to add a small handful of dulse or other
sea vegetable, in which case leave out the tamari and add a little filtered
water as necessary to blend.

....

Tastied Sesame Seeds
(Protein rich)

I would miss toasted sesame seeds if I did not have these. I make plenty
and keep them in a jar ready for use. By soaking the sesame seeds, and
sprouting them for 24 hours if possible to bring them back to life, and
then dehydrating them you create something like toasted sesame seeds,
without damaging the seeds and zapping the nutrition. I make them
plain and with tamari.

1 cup soaked sesame seeds
Optional: 1 tablespoon tamari

Mix the tamari in well and spread the seeds out on a silicone sheet in a dehydrator, in sunshine or in an airing cupboard, until they are completely dry, perhaps in a couple of hours.

Sprinkle over savoury dishes and salads, either as they are or crushed lightly just before use to release the flavour. Left whole, they keep well in an airtight container.

● ●

Corn Bread
(Carbohydrate rich)

This is good plain chewy bread.

6 cups fresh corn scraped from the cobs, or fresh frozen organic corn, defrosted.	Optional: 1 level teaspoon cumin seeds or caraway seeds
½ cup flax seeds/linseed	¼ cup cold pressed olive oil
2 level teaspoons coriander seeds	½ cup filtered water
	1 tablespoon tamari

Grind the flax and coriander seeds together till quite finely ground. Add the cumin or caraway seeds and pulse briefly to break them up a little. Process all the other ingredients together until reasonably smooth, but still with some texture to the sweetcorn. Add the flax mixture and process to mix.

Spread it over two non-stick drying sheets and pat each half into a rectangle about ½ inch/1 centimetre thick with a spatula. Score each rectangle lightly into large squares. Dehydrate for a few hours until pleasantly chewy, timing things so that you can keep an eye on them towards the end, and not let them get too dry.

Essene Bread
(Carbohydrate rich)

The Essenes lived in the Middle East around the time of the Christ. As far as we know, they ate sprouted seeds and grains, and made flat bread by drying sprouted grain in the sun. If you live somewhere hot and dry enough you could try it that way. Otherwise, here is a dehydrator version.

¼ cup flax seeds/linseed
¼ cup filtered water + ¾ cup water
½ teaspoon caraway seeds
1 teaspoon sea salt
2½ cups sprouted wheat (measured when just starting to sprout)
1 tablespoon cold pressed olive oil

Soak the flax seed in ¼ cup filtered water while preparing the rest of the dough. Put the rest of the ingredients in a food processor and process until a dough is formed which looks smooth overall but is still very grainy. Add the soaked flax seeds and process for a couple of seconds to mix.

Spread into ovals like small pita bread about ½ centimetre/ ¼ inch thick on non-stick drying sheets. Dehydrate for an hour or more, lift off the drying sheets onto the mesh tray, and dry a little further until chewy and firm but not dry.

Salad Dressing Flakes for Travelling
(Protein rich)

Who knows what salad dressings you may be offered when eating out. I have heard the suggestion that you take your own raw dressing with you, but I have not wanted to risk a bag full of leaked dressing or to be that much of a fuss-pot in public. Then I had a 'eureka!' moment. I thought I could dehydrate a dressing into little flakes to spread over restaurant salad. Then, to make it moist, I could surreptitiously tip a little water from my glass over the salad. It works, and here it is:

1 cup soaked sunflower seeds	powder or ground mustard
¼ cup Mila/ground chia seeds	seeds
4 tablespoons tamari	1 large clove garlic
6 tablespoons lemon juice	6 tablespoons cold pressed olive
1 tablespoon prepared mustard,	oil
less if it is a hot mustard, or a	Optional: ¼ teaspoon cayenne
pinch or two of mustard	pepper

Blend or process the sunflower seeds with everything except the chia seeds/Mila and blend to a smooth cream. If using a blender, tip the mixture into a bowl and stir in the Mila/ground chia seeds. If using a processor, just add the Mila/chia and process to mix it in.

Spread the mixture as thinly as possible over 4-5 non-stick drying sheets. Dehydrate for a few hours until completely crisp and store in an airtight container. Then, take some out with you in a tiny container, order some plain salad, sprinkle it over the top and, hey presto, you have a meal.

I did this to test the recipe, and ordered plain salad and plain steamed vegetables. It tasted great and my companions were a touch envious.

Crunchy Ginger Walnuts
(Protein rich)

These irresistible spiced walnuts are for snacking and parties.

2 cups walnuts, revived and de-bittered by soaking and rinsing, then
  dehydrated before you start this recipe
Optional (I like these a little sweet): I teaspoon of honey or a tiny
  spoon/drop of pure stevia extract
I small or medium carrot
I chunk peeled fresh ginger, the size of two Brazil nuts
½ teaspoon herb salt or a few splashes of tamari
2 tablespoons cold pressed olive oil
2 tablespoons filtered water
2 teaspoons ground chia seeds/Mila

Blend everything together except the chia/Mila and the walnuts and
blend to a thick cream. Add the chia/Mila and blend briefly to mix.

Put the walnuts in a large bowl. Add the blended ingredients and
massage in with your hands to cover the nuts evenly. Spread on mesh
dehydrator trays and dehydrate all day or overnight until crunchy.

You could vary the recipe by adding a little garlic and blending in fresh
herbs instead of the ginger.

Browned Onions

A delicious way with onions is to marinate them in the minimum of oil and modest splashes of tamari, and then to soften them in a dehydrator. Slice them thinly, lengthwise for oriental meals and crosswise for European meals. Leave them in the dehydrator for a shorter or longer time depending on how you like them. Dry them for a couple of hours for a 'stir-fry' texture, longer for a more chewy texture.

···

Marinated Shitake Mushrooms

These marinated mushrooms are delightful mixed into salads and oriental dishes. They are wonderful in wraps and nori rolls, and perfect in a **'Full British'** breakfast

2 cups shitake mushrooms, minus the tough stems, pressed into the cup.
1-2 tablespoons cold pressed olive oil
1 tablespoon tamari

Stir the ingredients together or massage them with your hands. Leave covered on the side for the flavours to mix. The flavour and texture of these outstandingly nutritious mushrooms is wonderful. They are delicious just like this, or you can dehydrate them for a couple of hours to develop the flavour and change the texture.

Crunchy Base for Pizza and Quiche
(Carbohydrate rich)

1 cup 'buckwheaties'
3 medium carrots
1 small mild red or white onion
1 tablespoon flax seed/linseed
1 teaspoon mixed herbs or Herbes de Provence
1 tablespoon tamari
A pinch of **Garlic Powder** or ½ a clove of garlic

Juice or blend the carrots, garlic and onion and mix the juice and fibre in a big bowl with the dry 'buckwheaties'. Grind the flax seeds and add in with the other ingredients. Stir it all well and leave to thicken for a few minutes. Mix again and spread on non-stick drying sheets in 6-7 individual pizza circles about 5 in/13 cm, or into one or two larger circles about ½ cm/¼ in thick. Dehydrate all day or over night until completely crisp. You can press this mixture over the base and up the sides of a non-stick cake tin with a push-up base. Dehydrate it in the same way and fill it with interesting vegetables and a thick creamy avocado sauce for a carbohydrate-rich quiche.

Chewy Base for Pizza
(Protein rich)

Sunflower and Flax Seed Pizza Base

This one is made from sunflower seeds and flax seeds and is very high in protein.

For a large pizza to serve up to four with a large salad along side:

1 cup flax seeds/linseed	basil, or 1 tablespoon finely
1 cup sunflower seeds –	chopped fresh herbs
preferably already soaked	1 clove garlic
overnight and dehydrated	½ a small mild onion
1 teaspoon dried Italian herbs	1 cup filtered water
such as oregano, thyme and	2 tablespoons tamari

Grind the flax seeds in small batches and put them in a large bowl. Do not worry if some of them remain whole. Grind the sunflower seeds without letting them turn into butter. Add to the bowl. Put the water, onion, garlic and tamari in a blender and blend for a minute or so. Add the herbs and pulse for a couple of seconds. Add the mixture to the ground sunflower and flax seeds and stir well.

Setting aside a couple of tablespoons of the mixture, spread the mixture out into one very large circle on a non-stick drying sheet. Put pieces of the extra dough in the corners of the tray, flattened to the same thickness as the pizza base. These are for testing. Dehydrate for an hour or two until firm enough to flip over and peel back the silicone sheet. Dehydrate further for a few hours until the mixture is dryish but still pleasantly chewy, in fact like a regular pizza base.

You can also spread the mixture out into a rectangle and score it into toast-sized slices to dehydrate for raw chewy 'toasted' bread.

Good Sweet Treats

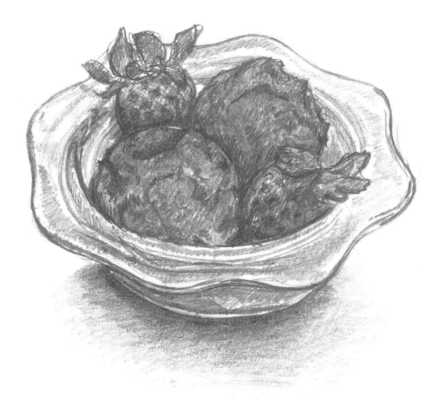

Fruit Sorbet

These treats are 'good' because they are a treat for your body as well as for your tastebuds. There are no potentially unhelpful ingredients and no food combining problems. That is unless you have decided, or been advised to, have no sugar at all, in which case there are still some treats in store for you here if you avoid the recipes that include fruit. Some of these treats are sweetened with stevia extract from the sweet-tasting but sugar-free stevia leaf. This is *not* the mixtures of stevia extract and other highly processed ingredients, some including sugar, that are now on sale in UK supermarkets. See **Good Resources** for sources of pure stevia extract. If you choose to sweeten any of the recipes with honey, agave syrup, maple syrup or yacon syrup then they will still be much much kinder to your system than regular sweet confections, but your body will have to deal with some sugar. The fruit treats of course contain the sugar in the fruit, which is why they are treats rather than everyday food. The nut treats would be rather rich to have every day.

Desserts are best served away from the main meal, but if you use pure stevia extract to sweeten a nut dessert you could serve it straight after a light salad and sprout meal and still have good protein-rich food combining.

Fruit Salads

Do not overlook the beauty and subtlety of the humble fruit salad. When I was growing up fruit salad always had orange segments, banana, grapes and apples. That is nice, but you can use your imagination. Fruit salads with just a couple of ingredients are very good. Try:

- Soft sliced pears and redcurrants
- Chopped sweet apples and blackcurrants
- Papaya and mangos
- Pineapple and peeled orange segments
- Bananas and pureed persimmon (In small servings because so sweet)
- Cherry purée over blueberries
- Pineapple pieces and slices of peeled orange

There are some magical ingredients for fruit salads. Passion fruit, with its divine juice and little pips, brings any fruit salad to life. A squeeze of lemon juice can make a difference, so can a little lemon zest, cinnamon powder, or vanilla essence. Try a grating of nutmeg, or a little powdered ginger or fresh ginger juice.

....

Melon Salad

Since melons are digested better on their own, for a special occasion make a pretty salad with different colours of chopped ripe melon. You can make melon balls with a gadget, piling up a mixture of two or three kinds in a serving bowl or in individual wine glasses. Ginger is the traditional flavouring, so perhaps add a little fresh ginger juice.

193

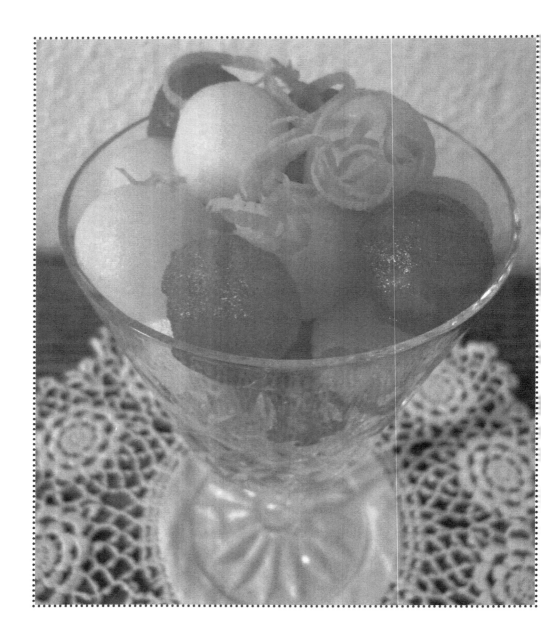

Melon Salad

Hippocrates Nut Icecream
(Protein rich)

This is the recipe for the delicious icecream they serve at Hippocrates on Saturday nights. People hang around waiting for icecream time because the word gets round that it is worth the wait. It probably stops people slipping away to find regular icecream.

About 11 cups nut milk made by:
soaking 2 cups walnuts and 2 cups pine nuts separately overnight. Rinse and discard the rinse and soak water. Blend 2 cups of filtered water with the walnuts and squeeze through a fine mesh bag. Repeat the process with the pine nuts in 2 cups filtered water. Alternating between the pine nuts and walnuts, add more water and squeeze out more milk until you have 11 cups.

To flavour add:

4 teaspoons cinnamon
Optional: 2+ teaspoons natural maple flavour (From the US)
1 whole vanilla pod or 2 tablespoons real vanilla essence, or more to
  taste
Pure stevia extract to taste

Flavour the milk to your liking, blending in the whole vanilla pod if you use one. Follow the instructions to make in an icecream maker (checking how much you can make at one time) or freeze hard in ice cube trays or other shallow containers and put the cubes through an auger juicer with the paté/mincing screen.

The maple flavouring adds something special but you could try almond essence, carob, or other natural flavourings.

Fruit Sorbet

This must be one of the easiest delicious and sophisticated fruit desserts, and there are three ways to make it.

1. Make it in your auger juicer. Freeze some clean, fresh, ripe fruit in chunks and put it through your juicer with the mincing/paté-making parts instead of the juicing parts. If you have an auger juicer such as the Omega or Oscar juicers you can do this, so get out the instruction book.
2. Make it in a powerful blender. Add small chunks of frozen fruit to the blender on quite a high speed, adding more as it starts to break down into sorbet. Do not try to make too much at once and do not wreck your blender by forcing it if it is not coping. You might need to leave the frozen fruit out of the fridge for a little while before you start. Put little bowls in the freezer beforehand so you can spoon the sorbet into freezing cold bowls.
3. Make sorbet in an ice-cream maker. Blend your chosen combination of fruit at room temperature and put the blended mixture in the ice cold ice-cream maker to make the sorbet.

Bananas on their own make the creamiest sorbet, almost like a soft-whip ice cream. Cut the bananas into chunks before freezing. A combination of berries, or a combination of tropical fruits, work well too. If you need to be very precise about food combining, do not mix the sweet bananas with the less sweet berries or tropical fruits.

If you make your sorbet in your juicer you can make rainbow sorbet, for example with yellow pineapple, orange mango, pink strawberries and purple black cherries.

Always use fresh, perfectly ripe fruit.

Festive Fruit Fool or Sorbet

This recipe needs a powerful blender.

2 sweet apples with their skins, cored and chopped
The insides of 3 passion fruit, including the seeds
A large handful each of frozen raspberries and frozen cherries
  without stones

If you try this in a standard blender you might not pulverise the seeds in the passion fruit and raspberries sufficiently to avoid 'grit' in the fool or sorbet. A powerful blender can grind it all to smoothness. You get the benefit of the nutrition inside the seeds and a good texture. Serves 3-4

Blend the apples and passion fruit till smooth, adding in the raspberries a few at a time to prevent it from getting too warm.

Blend for long enough to get rid of the all the seeds. Add the cherries, blend briefly till just smooth, and serve it straight away as an ice-cold fool, or pour into an ice cream maker to freeze for sorbet.

This is an exceptionally nice flavour combination, but experiment and I am sure you will come up with other good combinations.

If you have a regular blender try something like cherries and peeled apples – no seeds to worry about.

· ·

Fruit Jelly

This might not be strong enough or wobbly enough to set it in an old-fashioned jelly mould, which is a pity, but it does set and it is very refreshing. You will need a powerful blender that can deal with the tiny fruit seeds and skins. Depending on how much pectin – which is the natural jelling agent – there is in the fruit, other combinations of fruit can work too. Serves 3-4.

2 teaspoons psyllium husks
1 cup raspberries
1 cup blueberries
1 apple, pips and tough bits removed but keeping the well washed skin

Blend all together till super smooth and pour into one large dish or 3-4 small dishes. Leave in the fridge for several hours. The raspberries pull the tastes together. I did not like it much until I added the raspberries, and then it was delicious.

....

Marmalade

The skins of oranges, limes and lemons have no sugar and neither does the juice of lemons and limes. Use whichever you like. I have made this with a mixture of ordinary oranges and a bitter Seville orange, and it is delicious to my special English bitter marmalade taste buds. If you use orange juice there will be a little sugar, but hardly enough to worry about since this is a conserve to spread thinly on dehydrated oatcakes, breads and crackers. The sweetness comes from pure stevia extract.

1 orange chopped and with the seeds removed (a Seville orange if you like very bitter marmalade)
The juice of a second orange
Pure stevia essence, powder or liquid

Blend the orange chunks and juice together and little by little add stevia until it is as incredibly sweet as regular jam or marmalade.

Scrape the mixture out and keep it in a jar in the fridge. It will set further in the fridge from the action of the pectin in the fruit.

If you wish, you can peel off some thin strands of orange zest from the skin before you start. Add them to the blended marmalade so that you have some fine peel in the finished marmalade. Mine only kept for about a week, so do not make too much at once. The same method is fine for lemons and limes, but you might need to add water as there may be less juice in proportion to the amount of pith and skin.

....

Lemon Curd

This is a rich spread that has sesame oil in it in place of the butter in regular lemon curd. It is quite similar to regular lemon curd. It is good on plain dehydrated crackers such as **Oatcakes**, or on **Essene bread**. It sets quite firmly in the fridge because of the pectin in the lemon and you could use a layer of it, perhaps with less stevia, in a fancy fruit dessert or over ice cream. The minute pinch of 'black' Himalayan salt, which is actually pink, rounds out the taste in an egg-like way, but it is not essential. The salt makes it more like conventional lemon curd, but is not essential either.

A small lemon or half a large one, minus the pips	¼ cup cold pressed sesame oil
1 tablespoon chia/Mila seeds	¼ cup filtered water
Optional: a pinch of sea salt.	Plenty of pure stevia extract
Optional: a minute pinch of black Himalayan salt	(Lemon curd is sweet, remember)

Cut the lemon into chunks and blend together everything except the stevia. Then add stevia a tiny spoon or a drop at a time until it is really quite sweet, as sweet as you like. Blend well and keep covered in the fridge.

199

Angel Pair Cream

A simple, creamy treat with just the sugar from the pears and a little stevia. The name is a pun on the two pear ingredients, regular pears and avocado pears. Serves 2.

1-2 perfectly ripe pears
½ a medium or large perfectly ripe avocado pear
A few drops or a tiny spoon of pure stevia extract
A squeeze of lemon juice

In a blender blend the pear to a thin puree. Add the chopped avocado and blend to a thick cream, adding stevia and lemon juice to taste as you wish. Serve in small bowls or glasses and decorate with slices or little pieces of pear (dipped in lemon juice to stop them turning brown).

··

Avocado Cream

While you can make fantastic nut creams that are so good you will not miss dairy cream, they are not the best food combination with fruit. Fruit with nut cream is a very nice decadence, but here is an everyday topping that is a good combination with fruit. The flavourings, and the dried fruit if you use it, distinguish it from the vanilla custard in the next recipe.

Make use of the fact that avocados combine well with fruit and the way avocado blends to a creamy texture to make a subtle creamy topping. Mulberries are getting easier to find. Try an Indian or Iranian delicatessen or a health food shop. The mulberries do go very well with the cinnamon and nutmeg, but if you cannot find them, dates are fine.

1 large handful dried mulberries or 2-3 fresh dates, or pure stevia
  extract to taste
½ a cup of filtered water
I large ripe avocado
A pinch of cinnamon
A small grating of fresh nutmeg

Soak the mulberries or dates in ½ cup water, more if necessary to cover.
Leave to soak for several hours.

Blend the mulberries or dates and the soak water together with the
spices. Add the avocado chunk at a time, and blend until smooth and
thick, adding a little more water as necessary for a consistency similar to
whipped cream. Or, blend the water and chopped avocado, adding stevia
a tiny spoon or drop at a time until it is sufficiently sweet. Serve with
fresh fruit salad.

••

Vanilla Custard

I agree, this custard is green rather than the usual colour for custard, but
it is pleasantly custardy to taste. You could serve it with chopped soft
ripe pears and travel right back to an English childhood. With children,
try calling it 'Shrek's custard'. Serves 4

1 medium-large avocado, peeled and chopped
1 tiny spoon or drop of pure stevia extract, or more to taste
1 teaspoon vanilla essence, or more to taste
Optional: a very tiny pinch of Himalayan black salt (for a hint of
  egg)
1½ cups filtered water, or more, depending on the size of the avocado

Mix all together in a blender and serve.

Banana Custard

This British childhood favourite tastes as good with raw **Vanilla Custard**, even if it is green. Keep the servings small because bananas are so sweet. Make custard from the previous recipe and add ripe banana slices. Stir them in. You can serve this cold, but to be traditional it is good warmed in the dehydrator. In that case, a skin will form, but when I was little that was part of the experience anyway.

....

Christmas Pudding Fruit Salad

I debated whether this delicious alternative to rich Christmas pudding, **Christmas Cake** and mince pies should go here or in the **Muddled Good Sweet Treats** chapter, because it is so sweet with the dried fruit.

The food combining is OK, even if you serve **Vanilla Custard** with it, so I slipped it in this chapter. To cut down on the sugar you can use less of the dried fruit and increase the amount of apples and pears, and still make a spiced Christmas fruit salad – or you can eat less.

5 apples and 5 perfectly ripe, not over ripe, pears, finely chopped	1 teaspoon finely grated fresh ginger
1 cup each of raisins (lexias if possible), sultanas and currants	1 teaspoon each finely grated orange and lemon zest
The juice of 3 oranges	The juice of ½ a lemon.
1 teaspoon cinnamon	

For a traditional British mixture of tastes, serve with **Vanilla Custard**.

Blueberry Cream

1 carton ripe blueberries
1 avocado
1 spoon of honey, 2 large fresh dates or a tiny spoon or drop of pure
stevia extract

Blend together the blueberries and avocado to a rich cream. Add your chosen sweetener a little at a time. Blend again and test the flavour.

It needs a touch of sweetness, but do not make it too sweet or you will lose the blueberry taste.

··

Mango Delight

Per person, blend together one very ripe sweet mango and half a ripe avocado. Add a little pure stevia extract to taste if you wish and blend again to mix it in. That is it.

You could decorate the serving bowl or bowls with a pattern of sliced mango, or add some chopped mango after blending. For a flan filling (which would muddle the food combining), add a little more avocado for a thicker cream.

This an exotic treat because it is important to wait for really ripe mangos. Nothing less than really ripe will do, for the taste or from a nutritional standpoint.

Carob Mousse

If you use stevia rather than honey or yacon, and almond milk rather than rice milk then these ingredients are good food combining. If you have any maca powder, try adding a teaspoonful to give a bitter, slightly chocolaty, edge to the taste.

½ cup Mila or chia seeds soaked in 2 cups of almond or rice milk
½ cup raw carob powder
¼ teaspoon cinnamon
1-2 teaspoons vanilla essence or a tiny spoon of powdered vanilla, or a couple of drops of maple essence
Optional: a tiny spoonful or drop of pure stevia extract or two teaspoons honey or yacon syrup
Optional: a pinch of sea salt

Blend the milk and Mila or chia seeds in a powerful blender until velvet smooth. Blend in the carob, cinnamon, vanilla and/or maple essence. Taste for sweetness. The carob is so sweet naturally that the mixture may be sufficiently sweet as it is, or add the stevia, honey or yacon syrup little by little. Serve straight away, or refrigerate for a thicker mousse.

Muddled Good
Sweet Treats

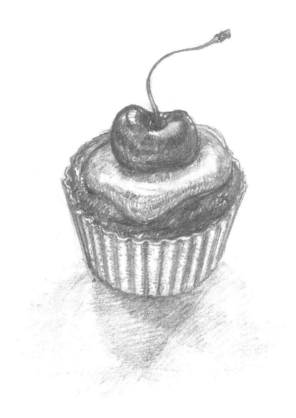

Carob Fruit Cup Cake

These are delectable all-raw treats for special occasions. They make no pretense at good food combining and most of them are rather sweet. That is why I have called them 'muddled' treats. They present the digestive system with a challenging mixture of foods and so create hard work. On one hand they are definitely a *vast* improvement on conventional sweets, such as those that fill supermarket aisles and cake shop windows, but they are much harder work for your system than the other recipes in this book.

You can see from the fact that there are quite a few recipes in this chapter that I do make them occasionally: *mea culpa* (which is Latin for 'my shortcoming').

Most I have dreamed up and made just once, for a special occasion or because inspiration struck. Many people find their way into the world of raw food through sweet treats, and if you are making a transition into raw foods and finding it tough, they can be an enjoyable occasional refuge.

As with the fruit dishes in the **Good Sweet Treats** section, if I were healing myself from something serious such as cancer or diabetes I would steer right round this section.

When I was going back and retesting the quantities in some recipes, I made a few in quick succession. It was only when I found I was hankering after chocolate when I was out, that my energy levels were less stable, and that I came down with a cough and a cold, that I clicked and made the connection between what was happening in my body and with eating too much sweet stuff! You have been warned.

Some of these muddled sweet treats call for coconut oil. It is raw, it is vegan and you can find organic. Opinions vary as to whether it is beneficial in nutritional terms because it is a saturated fat, and for that reason I only use it very occasionally. Make sure what you buy is not rancid. It goes rancid quickly and can start to taste unpleasantly like soap. If it tastes like that when you buy it, take it back. However, it can be a helpful ingredient for setting things and adding a lovely creamy taste.

I use a little salt in a few sweet recipes – tamari just would not work in sweet dishes! A little salt can round out flavours, but if you leave it out your sweet treats will still be treats.

I occasionally use cashew nuts for quick smooth creamy results, but only raw ones (see the **Good Ingredients** section on **Nuts and Seeds**) You can always use other soaked nuts such as pine nuts, pecan nuts and walnuts instead.

There are two recipes here for the raw sweet treats I showed on Television. These are the **Carob and Fruit Cupcakes** I made for pop star Lulu on *The Hour* on Scottish Television, and the **Raspberry and Hazelnut Cream Tart** that I got into the first round of the TV competition *Britain's Best Dish* – the first raw dish ever to get into the competition.

Enjoy these sweet treats that are so much better than conventional sweet 'food', *but* do make *much* more room on your table for delicious nutritious raw and living food vegan meals. Those are a joy to eat and you can get up from the table with plenty of energy for life. That is the real treat.

Date and Almond Butter Fridge Fudge

This is very sweet, but nowhere near as sweet as ordinary fudge. The deliciousness takes away any lingering wistfulness for traditional fudge.

3 large fresh Medjool dates
2 tablespoons cold pressed coconut oil at room temperature
A pinch of sea salt
½ teaspoon vanilla essence
3 tablespoons almond butter

In a food processor blend together everything except the almond butter until smooth and creamy. Add the almond butter and blend until even more creamy.

Pour into a shallow container such as an icecube tray in a 1centimetre/½ inch layer. Leave it to set in the fridge for several hours.

Cut into small squares and serve from the fridge.

....

Brazil Nut Fudge

½ cup cold pressed coconut oil
½ cup Yacon root powder or raw carob powder
½ cup chopped Brazil nuts
A pinch of sea salt
½ teaspoon vanilla essence and/or a few drops of natural maple
  flavour

Melt the oil over a turned-off cooled hot plate or in a double saucepan over warm, not boiling, water, and stir in the yacon or carob powder. Add vanilla, natural maple flavour and salt to taste and mix well. Stir in the Brazil nut pieces. Spoon into chocolate moulds or ice cream trays and pat down. Alternatively, leave out the chopped Brazil nuts and put a whole Brazil nut in each piece. Freeze and serve chilled.

Almond and Poppy Seed Treats

1 cup poppy seeds
Filtered water
1 cup fresh dates, stoned and pressed into the cup
2 cups of almonds, ideally soaked and dehydrated
½ vanilla pod
A pinch of sea salt
½ teaspoon each lemon and orange zest
1 cup soft raisins or sultanas

Soak the poppy seeds for several hours. Rinse, drain and leave to dry, or dehydrate briefly.

Grind the vanilla, almonds and salt in a food processor and add the dates a few at a time to form a dough. Transfer to a large bowl and mix in the lemon and orange zest well. Mix in the poppy seeds and raisins or sultanas, and knead briefly to a thick dough. Form into balls or press into little silicone cupcake cases.

Valentines Carob Fudge with Strawberries

This is pleasantly sweet and chewy. The carob, the coconut oil and the cinnamon sweeten it. The maca powder is not essential but it adds a bitter edge to the carob so that it is more like chocolate, but these are so good that you will not miss chocolate.

½ a cup of raw carob powder
½ a cup of cold pressed coconut oil at room temperature
A pinch of cinnamon
½ teaspoon of vanilla essence
1 teaspoon maca powder, optional
Dehydrated strawberry slices to decorate

For the strawberry slices, slice some well-shaped ripe strawberries lengthwise to reveal the heart shape. Lay the slices out carefully on a dehydrator tray – you do not need a non-stick drying sheet – and dehydrate for an hour or more so that they are dry on the outside but still slightly soft and moist.

Make the fudge by melting the coconut oil in a double saucepan over warm, not boiling, water, or over an electric hotplate that has been turned off and allowed to cool. When the coconut oil has melted, stir in the carob powder, cinnamon, vanilla and optional maca. Pour the mixture into silicone chocolate moulds, little silicone cup cake cases or ice cube trays. Decorate each piece with a slice of dried strawberry, gently pushing it onto the surface of the mixture. Put the fudge pieces in the fridge to set and serve them from the fridge or an insulated container.

Date, Vanilla and Sesame Halva

1 cup soaked and dehydrated sesame seeds
Optional: a pinch of sea salt
1 teaspoon vanilla essence
About 5 fresh dates, Medjool dates if possible.

Add the sesame seeds, salt and vanilla to a processor and process until most or all of the seeds are crushed.

Add the dates one at a time until it is sweet enough for your taste and the dough is well mixed.

Press the mixture down into an ice cube tray or similar and score into small pieces. Keep in the fridge to harden, and serve straight from the fridge.

....

Carob Iced Orange Creams

These little confections do not know whether they are desserts or smart confectionery. The crusts turn them into dinner party fare. It is good that they are small because they are so sweet. They are best served a while after dinner. Make them in tiny silicone cupcake cases. It does not work in paper cupcake cases because they collapse. The mixture is too runny until it sets in the freezer. The avocado does turn them a little green, even with the orange zest and juice. You could try lime instead and then that would not matter. Makes about a dozen.

Cream

2 medium avocados
3 tablespoons cold pressed coconut oil
1 heaped teaspoon orange zest
The juice of 1½ medium oranges
3 tablespoons honey or agave syrup or stevia to taste
Optional: A pinch of sea salt

Blend all the ingredients except one of the avocados until everything is smooth. Then add the second avocado in chunks and blend it in to thicken. Fill the little cup cake cases, leaving a little space at the top for the carob crust.

Crusts

¼ cup cold pressed coconut oil
¼ cup raw carob powder
Optional: 2 teaspoons raw maca powder

Melt the coconut oil in a saucepan on a hotplate that has been turned off and allowed to cool a little, or in a double saucepan over warm, not boiling, water. Stir the crust ingredients together and spread a little over each cupcake case. Freeze and serve from the freezer. Allow them to sit on the table in front of everyone for a few minutes before eating them, so that the cream can soften slightly.

Easy Trifle 'Messes'

This is a rich dessert faintly similar to Eton Mess because of the mixture of stirred-up cream and fruit colours. I like it this way. Serves 4

½ cup of macadamia nuts
2 tablespoons cold pressed coconut oil at room temperature
4 fresh dates, preferably Medjool dates
1 cup raspberries (frozen)
1 cup blueberries (frozen)
Optional: a pinch of sea salt
1 teaspoon vanilla essence
Filtered water

Soak the nuts and process with the coconut oil and the pitted dates with the minimum of water – a tablespoon or two – to a thick cream. Blend in the vanilla and the salt.

Turn the cream into a bowl. Add the frozen fruit and stir well. The frozen fruit thickens everything quickly.

Put spoonfuls into small silicone cupcake cases and serve. If you need to make these ahead of time, put them in the freezer to keep and then put them in the fridge an hour or so before you eat.

Serve with teaspoons.

Raspberry Jam

This is for decadent afternoon tea, spread on raw **Oatcakes** with **Butter Spread**. Or use it on cake or between cake layers.

Mix a cup of ripe raspberries with a little honey or agave syrup to taste, perhaps two teaspoons.

Spread the mixture out in a dish and dehydrate it for several hours until reduced in quantity with a syrupy juice. If necessary mix in a little more honey or agave.

You can refrigerate it to further thicken it, but serve it at room temperature for a more pronounced sweet raspberry taste.

Try this with blended cherries instead. It would go well on a carob cake, and in the **Carob and Cherry Black Forest Cake.**

. . . .

Rich Vanilla Custard

This is wonderful with the **Christmas Fruit Salad.** You could also make a Christmas pudding from the **Christmas Cake** recipe. If so, stir in a silver sixpence or traditional silver Christmas pudding charms for lucky people to find, and put the mixture in a traditional pudding bowl lined with cling-film so that you can lift it out and upend it to serve with a sprig of holly in the middle – and some of this divine custard. Serves 4

1 cup pine nuts or cashew nuts	A pinch of sea salt or black
1 cup walnuts	Himalayan salt
½ cup agave syrup, honey or	½ cup cold pressed coconut oil
maple syrup	at room temperature
Seeds from a vanilla pod	½ an avocado
	1 cup filtered water

Soak the nuts in cool water for a few hours and drain them. Blend the soaked nuts, cup of water, salt, coconut oil, vanilla and honey/maple/agave syrup in a powerful blender or processor. Then blend in the avocado. Refrigerate to thicken before serving.

....

Orange and Walnut Cream

This is a lovely, creamy nut dessert that you can serve as it is, with peeled fresh orange segments or as the filling in a flan case such as the Brazil nut flan case in the next recipe.

½ cup walnuts
3 large fresh raw dates such as Medjool dates
½ an avocado
Finely-grated zest from 1 orange
Juice of two oranges
1 tablespoon cold pressed coconut oil

Soak the walnuts for a few hours or overnight and rinse well. Soak a while longer and rinse again. The extra soak and rinse is to make sure the walnuts are de-bittered.

Blend together everything in a blender or processor except the avocado. Add the avocado in small chunks and blend again without stop/starting the blender. Set all day or overnight in the fridge.

Angelic Orange Cream

When you want something sweet, naughty, creamy and quick, and do not want to resort to anything whipped up from a packet of suspicious chemicals, or spooned from a plastic tub destined for landfill after a short life, try this. It is just right, richly flavoured but not over sweet and it does not have a lingering chemical aftertaste. In the marmalade-making season, try making it with part Seville bitter orange juice. Serves 2

1 avocado	3 tablespoons
2 tablespoons cold pressed	honey/yacon/agave or 2 tiny
coconut oil	spoons or drops of pure stevia
Grated peel from ¼ medium	extract
orange	The juice of 1½ medium
2 tablespoons water	oranges

Blend all together in a blender or food processor and put into small bowls. Refrigerate for several hours to chill and thicken, or eat it straight away!

....

Mandarin and Walnut Ice Cream

The juice of about 8 mandarins	Pure stevia extract powder or
A few strips of mandarin skin.	drops to taste
1 cup walnuts that have been	The seeds scraped from inside ½
soaked and dehydrated	a vanilla pod

Blend everything together and adjust the flavours to taste. Pure stevia extract seems to work very well in ice cream. Freeze in an ice cream maker and serve. Or, freeze in ice cube trays and put the frozen cubes through an auger juicer with the paté attachment, as for making **Sorbet**.

....

Lemon Torte

This is very easy, but still fancy enough to impress visitors. The lemon taste is fresh and on the bitter side so it is quite a sophisticated dessert. You could leave out the dates and add stevia so that it is sugar-free

Pastry crust

2 cups Brazil nuts
A generous pinch of sea salt

Grind or process the nuts and salt together until it is barely sticky enough to stick together and still has a slightly gritty texture (too far, and it goes like nut butter).

Knead into a ball of dough.

Press the dough down into the base of a pie dish, flat-based traditional soup plate or similar about 8 – 9inch/22centimetres across, working the dough up the sides high enough to pour in the filling and still show some pastry. You can fork the top edge as a decoration. Put the crust in the fridge to harden.

Lemon filling

2 large lemons or 3 small
2 large or 3 small avocados
1 cup pitted fresh raw dates
Filtered water

Use a blender or food processor. If your raw dates are dried, soak them in a little water overnight first. If any soak water remains, add that to the mixture.

Cut the lemons into eighths and blend the chunks, date soak water, and dates until smooth.

Cut the avocado into chunks and blend it in to the filling mixture. Keep adding chunks while keeping the blender going, so you can get a thicker mixture before it gets too thick for the blades to turn.

Add water little by little if necessary, remembering that you want a very thick creamy filling. Or, if the motor and blades cannot cope, mash the second half of the avocado to complete smoothness separately, and stir it in.

Spoon the mixture into a bowl, stir well and put the bowl in the fridge to thicken further.

Just before serving, spread the lemon filling in the pastry crust. Decorate with a few gratings or thin shavings of lemon zest.

. . . .

Vanilla and Almond Cake with Walnut and Honey Icing

Cake

½ cup almonds, soaked, skinned and dehydrated or ½ cup ground
  almonds
½ cup whole chia seeds
½ cup tightly packed dates
½ a cup of filtered water
2 teaspoons vanilla
½ cup poppy seeds
Optional: a pinch of sea salt

Soak the poppy seeds in water for an hour. Grind the almonds finely and place in a mixing bowl.

Put the water and dates in a blender or small processor bowl and blend or process until smooth.

Add the vanilla and salt and blend for another couple of seconds.

Add the mixture to the almonds and stir well. Drain the poppy seeds and stir them into the almond and date mixture. Add the chia seeds and stir all together to form a smooth dough. Pat the mixture into a small serving dish and leave at room temperature for a while for the chia seeds to soak up the excess moisture from the water in the dough.

Spread with the icing and refrigerate till time to serve.

Walnut and Honey Icing

A pinch of sea salt
1 cup walnuts, soaked and rinsed
2 teaspoons of honey
1 tablespoon cold pressed coconut oil at room temperature
Filtered water as necessary

Grind the walnuts with a little water to a smooth thick cream, adding the honey, salt and coconut oil. Blend till as smooth as possible, adding more honey to taste. Spread over the cake and refrigerate for several hours to set.

To avoid the coconut oil in the icing, substitute with half a small avocado.

Café Glazed Orange and Almond Cake

In the interests of science, I had a large slice of gluten-free orange and almond cake in a very nice Auckland café, and later came up with this raw version. It is not as sweet, but the honey taste goes further than agave syrup would. If you want a non-sweet, non-acidic version you could make a lemon and pure stevia extract version with some orange peel zest in it and then it would just about qualify for the **Good Sweet Treats** section.

Cake

½ cup chia seeds/Mila
3 ½ cups orange juice
Zest of ½ – ¾ an orange
1 cup macadamia nuts
3 tablespoons cold pressed honey
A very tiny spoon of black Himalayan salt (for the egg taste)
4 cups ground almonds
3 tablespoons cold pressed coconut oil at room temperature

Chop the macadamia nuts roughly and leave to soak in water for several hours. Process the chia seeds to crush them a little and leave them or the Mila to soak in 1 cup orange juice.

Rinse and drain the macadamia nuts and grind in a processor until sandy. Add the two remaining cups of orange juice and blend to a cream. It does not matter if it is still a little grainy.

Blend in the coconut butter. Stir the chia/Mila and juice mixture with the macadamia cream in a mixing bowl and add the orange zest and the tiniest pinch of black Himalayan salt. Add the honey and stir in well.

Lastly, stir in the ground almonds and press the mixture into an 8inch/20centimetre small spring-form cake tin or tin with a push-up base.

Leave to set in the fridge for half a day, or in the freezer for an hour and then back to the fridge till serving time.

Orange and Honey Glaze

1 teaspoon orange zest
2 teaspoons honey
2 teaspoons orange juice

Mix all together and leave to marinate in the fridge while the cake sets. Drizzle, drip or spread over the orange and almond cake before serving.

. . . .

Carob Birthday Cake

This is a good solid dark rich cake, which you can ice and serve with **Pouring Cream.** The cake also appears in the next recipe as a layered **Carob and Cherry Black Forest Cake**.

Carob Cake

1 cup ground almonds (ideally soaked, skinned, dehydrated and
   freshly ground, or simply buy organic ground almonds!)
½ cup whole chia seeds soaked in 1 cup filtered water
3 tablespoons cold pressed coconut oil at room temperature
½ cup fresh dates, stones removed, soaked in ½ cup filtered water
½ cup carob powder
1 teaspoon vanilla essence
1 pinch sea salt

If the coconut oil is solid, melt it in a saucepan that has been full of hot water or on a hotplate that has been turned off and allowed to cool a little.

221

Process the soaked dates and any soak water with the coconut oil, vanilla essence and sea salt.

Add the soaked chia seeds/Mila and lastly the carob powder and almonds. It may all form into well-mixed dough, or you may have to scrape it all out into a big bowl and mix it further with a wooden spoon.

Press the mixture into a non-stick cake tin with a push-up base. For softer brownies you can leave out the coconut oil.

Carob Icing

1 cup fresh dates, soaked in a little filtered water until soft
½ cup cold pressed coconut oil at room temperature
1 – 2 teaspoons vanilla essence or the seeds from a vanilla pod
½ cup carob powder
½ cup cashew nuts or macadamia nuts, soaked
Optional: a tiny pinch of sea salt

Process everything except the carob powder together in a food processor. Add the carob powder a spoon at a time until the icing is well-mixed, adding a little more water if necessary. Spread over the top, or, more thinly, over the top and the sides of the cake and refrigerate to harden further.

If you put the mixture in icecream trays or little chocolate moulds it makes good carob fudge

Pouring Cream

This is good with any kind of cake. It is rich from the nuts, but not too sweet. Serve separately in a jug

½ cup pecan nuts
½ cup pine nuts or cashew nuts
2 teaspoons lemon juice
Optional: a pinch of salt
2 tablespoons honey/maple syrup/agave syrup or 2 tiny spoons or
  drops of stevia
1-2 teaspoons vanilla extract
1 cup filtered water

Blend everything together for a rich pouring cream.

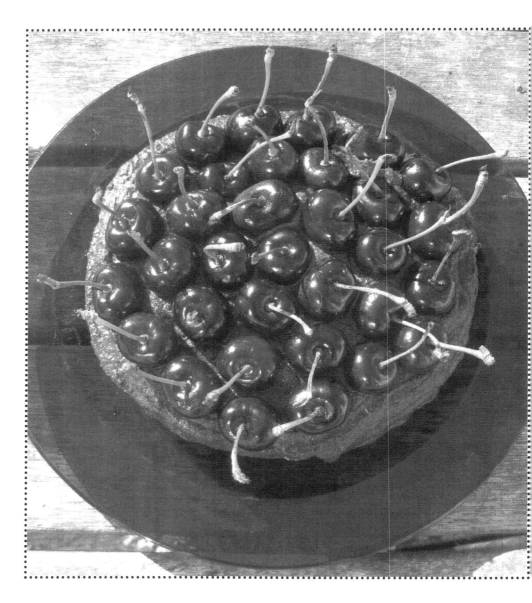

Carob Cherry Black Forest Cake

Carob Cherry Black Forest Cake

This is twice as tall as the **Birthday Cake**, or you could make it in a single, bigger cake tin and pile on the toppings.

Double the ingredients with a carton or two of ripe black cherries. Reserve enough whole cherries with their stalks to cover the whole of the top of the cake.

Make a thick sweet **Cherry Jam** with the rest of the cherries by removing the pips and blending them with fresh dates.

Cake

Double the **Birthday Cake** quantities and make 2 same size circles, each 2 centimetres/1inch thick in two non-stick cake tins with push up bases. Let the cakes harden in the fridge overnight or for a few hours.

Fillings:

Cherry Jam, as above, and double the quantity of **Carob Icing**.

Assembly

Put 1 cake on a serving dish. Spread it with a layer of cherry jam and a layer of half the icing. Carefully lift the second cake with two fish slices and place it on the icing layer. Use the rest of the icing to ice the top of the cake, smoothing it down the sides if you wish. Press whole black cherries with their stalks up all over the top of the cake (a black cherry stalk forest :-) and refrigerate to thicken the icing.

Serve with **Pouring Cream**, as above.

Apple Crumble

This English pudding manages to be quite sweet enough just from the apples and the tiny mount of honey or stevia. Try serving it with **Vanilla Custard** to bring back childhood memories. Serves 4-6

6-8 sweet apples, depending on size
2 cloves or a large pinch of powdered cloves
1 cup 'buckwheaties', (dehydrated sprouted buckwheat)
A pinch of sea salt
2 teaspoons honey or agave syrup, or 2 teaspoons filtered water + a
  few drops or a tiny spoon of pure stevia extract
3 tablespoons cold pressed coconut oil at room temperature
2 teaspoons filtered water
Cinnamon powder to sprinkle over the top

Melt the coconut oil over a bowl of hot water, or in a saucepan on a hotplate that has been turned off and allowed to cool down, and mix with the honey, salt and water in a bowl. Grind the 'buckwheaties' into flour. Add the flour to the coconut oil mixture and rub in well. Press down into the bowl and put in the fridge to harden as the coconut oil sets.

Meanwhile, peel and core the apples and chop them roughly. Grind the cloves and put them in a food processor with the apple. Process to a rough puree with little lumps of apple left in it. Spread the apple mixture into a suitable dish such as a traditional pie dish.

Bring the hardened crumble mixture out of the fridge and break it into rough chunks and crumbs, digging in with a knife or spoon. Spread the crumble over the apple and pat down gently. Sprinkle lightly with cinnamon to 'brown' it and to add a sweet taste. Return the crumble to the fridge until ready to serve.

Christmas Cake or Wedding Cake

This is a rich, moist, traditional fruitcake that can be iced with **Date Almond Paste** in the traditional way. It looks beautiful that way and you can make little decorations out of the almond paste (like marzipan but less sweet), and if you want a white surface you can grind a teaspoon or two of ordinary white sugar to make 'icing sugar' to sprinkle over the almond paste. Put the ground sugar in a sieve and shake it over the cake until there is just enough to colour the surface. For a wedding cake, decorate with edible flowers such as wild pansies or violets, rose petals, rose buds and roses in bloom.

¾ cup each of currants, raisins and sultanas
¾ cup chopped fresh dates
½ teaspoon each of lemon and orange zest
1¼ cups orange juice
¼ cup lemon juice
2 pinches vanilla powder or 1-2 teaspoons vanilla essence
1 ½ cups ground almonds
½ cup chia seeds/Mila
½ teaspoon ground cinnamon
1 teaspoon finely-grated fresh ginger
A light grating of nutmeg
3 tablespoons cold pressed walnut oil
I tablespoon of carob powder (to darken the mixture for authenticity)

Soak the dried fruit, lemon and orange zest, and spices all day or overnight in a large mixing bowl. Stir in the chia/Mila, the oil, the carob and the ground almonds, making Christmas wishes as you stir. Press the mixture into a silicone non-stick cake pan with a base that pushes up or that has a spring-form side opening. Leave to harden a little in the fridge before icing with **Date Almond Paste**.

Date Almond Paste or Marzipan

The traditional way with a fruitcake for Christmas or a wedding cake is to ice it in almond paste/marzipan. To ice the cake with the paste use less dates so that it is not too sweet. For marzipan for making little marzipan sweets you can add more dates. The traditional recipes have a lot of sugar in them. This recipe has fresh dates instead and is far less sweet, even though it is quite sweet enough to compete with the dried fruit in the cake.

2½ cups of ground almonds (not soaked)
½ – ¾ cup of fresh raw dates ideally the soft Medjool variety (½ a
   cup for almond paste or ¾ cup for marzipan)
1-2 teaspoons vanilla essence
2-4 teaspoons lemon juice

For almond paste use ½ cup of dates, removing the stones and tightly packing them into the measuring cup.

Put the dates in a food processor with a couple of spoons of the ground almonds. Process to a sandy consistency, and spoon by spoon add the rest of the ground almonds.

Before the mixture starts to clump together, add the vanilla and half the lemon juice and process a little further.

Taste and add more lemon if you wish. Process until the mixture forms a solid lump. Roll it out with a rolling pin to form a large circle, quite a bit larger than the cake.

Cut an exact circle from the mixture, slightly larger than the cake. Put it on top of the cake. Roll the rest of the paste up again and roll it out into a long narrow strip, the height of the cake in width. Use this strip to put a band of paste all around the cake to cover it completely. Gently roll again on the sides and top to get a good even shape. Decorate with whole blanched almonds or shake a little icing sugar or ground table sugar over the top through a sieve.

To make marzipan for sweets and decorative shapes use ¾ cup of dates and make in the same way as the almond paste.

Add a little carob powder to half of the mixture and mix it in well so that you have two different colours to play with.

···

Carob and Fruit Cupcakes

These are the raspberry cupcakes I made for popstar Lulu on TV, or you can make them with cherries or stawberries. She approved, as you can see on my website. The recipe makes about 16 cupcakes in mini-silicone cupcake cases. These days I would do things slightly differently. I would replace the coconut oil and lecithin in the carob cake mixture with ½ cup of cold pressed sesame oil and and two teaspoons of Mila or ground chia seeds. I would replace the coconut oil and lecithin in the raspberry icing with two teaspoons of psyllium husks. I would also use a mixture of soaked pine nuts and pecan nuts, or all pine nuts, instead of the cashew nuts.

Cake mixture:

¾ cup soaked almonds
½ cup tightly packed with fresh dates + 4 more dates
¼ cup cold pressed coconut oil
½ cup Brazil nuts, not soaked
½ cup carob powder
¼ teaspoon sea salt
½ a vanilla pod or 3 teaspoons of vanilla essence

Add the Brazil nuts to the food processor with the vanilla pod and process into small grains – too far and you will get nut butter. Add the carob powder and process further until it is quite a fine flour, but stop before it starts clumping. Tip the mixture into a bowl.

Warm the coconut oil over very warm water. Remove the stones from the dates and put them in the food processor with the coconut butter. Process till it forms a thick smooth batter.

Add the Brazil nut/carob 'flour' and process for a few seconds to mix.

Press the mixture lightly into little silicone cupcake cases and fill ¾ full.

Raspberry (or other fruit) Cream Icing:

1 ½ cups soaked cashew nuts
1 ½ cups raspberries + some raspberries left whole for decoration (or cherries or strawberries)
½ cup agave syrup.
¼ cup almond milk (made by blending half a cup of soaked almonds to a cup of filtered water and straining through a fine sieve)
1 tablespoon lemon juice
A pinch of sea salt
4 teaspoons vanilla essence
½ cup cold pressed coconut oil
1 tablespoon soy lecithin

Add everything to your blender except the coconut oil and lecithin and blend till very smooth and creamy. Stop blending and add the lecithin and coconut oil. Blend again until the oil and lecithin are mixed in completely. Leave the icing to set in the fridge.

Using a whipped cream/icing star nozzle, spoon the set icing into an icing bag and swirl round the cakes, covering the whole of each one. Decorate with a fruit on each cupcake and leave to firm again in the fridge.

Raspberry and Hazelnut Cream Tart

This is the recipe that made it into the first round of Britain's Best Dish TV competition, the first raw recipe to be accepted on the show. I had to make it in a fixed time, hence taking it in and out of the freezer. You only need to do that if you are in a hurry. It is a labour of love for a very special occasion. You can leave the coulis step out if you just want to put the tart on the table and serve slices right there, which you probably do want to do. You will need an 8inch /20centimetre non-stick sponge tin with a push-out base

Hazelnut pastry:

3½ cups of raw hazelnuts
A large pinch of sea salt

¼ cup cold pressed coconut oil
at room temperature
3 fresh Medjool dates

Creamy Vanilla filling:

1½ cups macadamia nuts
The seeds and soft scrapings out
of a vanilla pod
10 fresh Medjool dates
1 tablespoon soy lecithin

½ cup cold pressed coconut oil
at room temperature
1 cup of water
A pinch of sea salt

Pear and Raspberry Puree:

3 ripe pears, peeled
¾ cup ripe raspberries

1 large Medjool date

Raspberry Decoration and Raspberry Coulis:

3 cups of ripe raspberries (those with the best shapes for the
  decoration, the rest for the coulis)
A few edible flowers such as wild pansies or violets

Process the hazelnuts, dates, coconut oil and salt for the pastry until finely ground and ready to squash together into a paste. Turn it out into a bowl and work till sufficiently sticky to use as pastry. Put one quarter aside. Press the rest into the sponge tin to form an even crust that comes up exactly to the top of the tin all round. Leave to set in the fridge.

Process the all ingredients for the filling until smooth. Spread thinly in a large dish and leave to set in the fridge for several hours.

Wash all the raspberries. Pick the best ones for decoration and gently pat them dry with kitchen paper. Set them aside.

Cut and peel the pears and blend them with the rest of the raspberries and the date to a thick smooth purée.

Fork through the semi-set cream filling and spread it evenly into the hazelnut crust. Smooth the fruit puree evenly over the cream, reserving a little to add to the coulis.

Picking the ones with the best shapes, gently press raspberries all over the fruit puree to completely cover it, keeping them upright and leaving a little space around the edge ready for the pastry diamond decoration. Place the tart back in the freezer while making the pastry decoration.

Knead the rest of the hazelnut pastry to soften it and roll it out to about ½centimetre /¼inch thick. Cut into strips about 2.5cm/1inch wide and across at an angle to form diamonds. Re-roll the scraps and keep cutting until you have at least 25 diamonds.

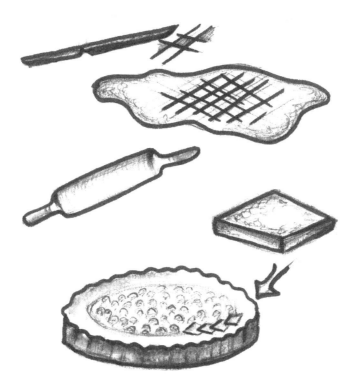

Bring out the tart and decorate the edge by overlapping the diamonds all round.

Place the tart back in the fridge.

Rub the raspberries for the coulis through a sieve and reserve the coulis.

To serve, place a slice on a plate and decorate the plate with the coulis and edible flowers.

Carrot Cake

As well as being English, I am a New Zealand citizen, and it would be practically illegal for me to write a recipe book with no Kiwi-style carrot cake recipe. This one is a worthy pioneering achievement in the tradition, with just the right mixture of carrot flavour, sweetness and slightly sour icing.

Decoration

Thin carrot slices cut into stars by hand or with a tiny cutter from a cook shop

Cake

2 cups carrot juice	½ cup Mila/ground chia
2 cups of carrot fibre from juicing	3 cups ground almonds
¾ cup of fresh dates, Medjool if possible	2 teaspoons of mixed spice
	Optional: ½ teaspoon of salt
2 Brazil-nut sized pieces of peeled ginger	2 teaspoons lemon juice

Soak the dates in the carrot juice until softened and process with the ginger to break down the ginger. Mix everything else in a large bowl and stir in the date mixture. Pat the mixture down in an 8inch/20centimetre non-stick push up or spring form cake tin and refrigerate until firm.

Icing

These quantities will ice the cake thinly. Double them for a thicker icing on the top and the sides of the cake.

½ cup of filtered water	Optional: ¼ teaspoon salt
4 tablespoons lemon juice	4 tablespoons of honey
1 cup pine nuts that have been	1 tablespoon psyllium hulls
soaked for several hours	1 teaspoon vanilla extract

Blend everything together and ice your cake. Decorate with carrot stars and impress your Kiwi friends.

Good Breakfasts

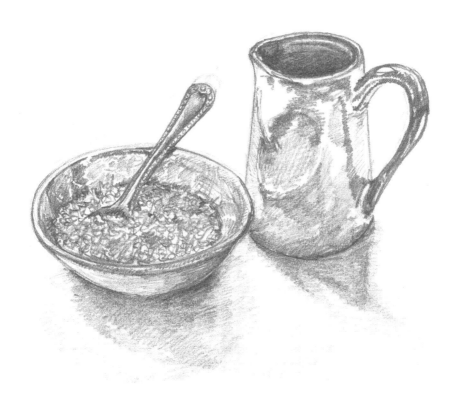

Buckwheaties cereal and oat milk

The word 'breakfast' is a good indication of what is happening in your system when you get up in the morning. It is still in fasting mode and so it is detoxing. You can allow the helpful detoxing process to continue a little longer by drinking lemon juice or herb tea before eating anything. That is preferable to drinking coffee or regular tea, either of which kick you roughly into the day with caffeine. Then it is time to break your fast gently with a large shot of **Wheatgrass Juice** and a little later **Green Juice** (see the **Good Drinks** section). That is the routine at the Hippocrates Health Institute in the mornings. Many people find the incredibly nourishing green juice is sufficient for breakfast. They save themselves for a big raw lunch later on. This has not worked for me, though perhaps it would have had I been living in a warmer climate. These are the kinds of breakfast I enjoy. They give me nourishment and sustenance for a busy morning.

Last Night's Dinner

I do not do this very often, but occasionally it feels right, and raw savouries and salads sitting and waiting in the fridge get finished off.

Fruit

This is served for breakfast about three times a week at the Hippocrates Health Institute. Melon, one kind alone or mixed with other varieties of melon only, is quick to digest and can make a good breakfast. I would rather have fruit occasionally as a treat or snack between meals, because it does not suit me for breakfast, presumably because of the sugar. Find out what works for you. It is certainly better to have plain fruit than to mix it into conventional muesli which mixes up fruit, nuts and grain flakes, usually not even soaked. Muesli is tough work for the digestive system, however delicious and filling it is.

Having said that about muesli, sometimes when faced with a hotel breakfast buffet with a long row of cooked dishes, toast and fruit, I select a very ripe banana and slice it into a 'porridge' of Mila and nut, rice or oat milk (I take along my own Mila sachets and a box of purchased nut or grain milk). The food combining is not the best, but at least the banana is raw and it is appetizing, and it is satisfying enough to keep me away from the wheat toast, baked beans and hash browns!

Buckwheaties

Make your own crunchy cereal in your dehydrator with sprouted buckwheat. Soak several cups of buckwheat overnight in a large mixing bowl.

Rinse off the thick liquid in a large sieve and soak for the day.

Drain, rinse and drain again, and leave the drained buckwheat seeds to sprout for a couple of days until tiny roots are starting to show, rinsing and draining again night and morning until they are ready.

Then spread them out on non-stick drying sheets and dehydrate for a few hours until they are completely dry and crisp. They keep well, so make plenty at a time if you like them. For a cereal breakfast, serve with oat, buckwheat, rice or quinoa milk, a tiny spoon or drop of pure stevia extract to sweeten, and perhaps a spoon of hemp oil for richness. You can make the milk by blending a little of the sprouted buckwheat or other grain with water, and a little good quality oil.

....

Oatmeal

Raw soaked oat flakes would be a great breakfast, if only it were easy to get raw oat flakes. You can find them online, see **Good Resources,** but most, probably all, in the shops are already steamed in the rolling process so they are not raw. If you have some cooked food or can get raw rolled oats, then rolled oat flakes soaked overnight and served with oat milk and pure stevia extract are a good simple breakfast.

Oat Porridge

Oats are a warming grain. I figure that since the organic flaked porridge oats you can buy in regular shops are already cooked it does not make a lot of difference if you turn them into cooked oat porridge, especially on an icy winter morning when you are going to have to wrap up warmly just to leave the house. I soak the oat flakes over night and then boil them in water in the traditional way. I like mine with oatmilk, sesame oil and pure stevia extract, sometimes with pollen, and even with a little powdered seaweed for saltiness and more nutrition. The rest of my meals would most probably be 100% raw that day.

....

Almond and Chia Seed Porridge

This is very rich and nourishing and I suggest you have just a small bowl.

Soak ¼ cup chia seeds or Mila in 1 cup almond milk overnight. Stir in ¼ cup ground almonds, a tiny spoon or drop of pure stevia extract and more almond milk to taste. Instead of, or as well as, the stevia, you can stir in a big spoonful of pollen for the all-round nutrition and sweet flowery taste.

Crackers, Butter Spread and...

Home made raw dehydrated oatcakes, corn chips, crackers and breads make a good breakfast, especially with **Butter Spread**. Why stop there? Add a pile of different sprouts to your plate and make open sandwiches.

Since there is negligible sugar in a little **Marmalade** or **Lemon Curd** when made to my recipes, you can have these for breakfast on dehydrated crackers, breads and **Oatcakes**, with or without a little **Butter Spread**.

....

A Favourite Savoury Breakfast

At the Hippocrates Health Institute some people have a small bowl of cooked grain-like seed for breakfast, either quinoa or millet, boiled gently. This became my favourite breakfast and it still is.

On the side there is always the same selection of healthy condiments – cold pressed olive oil, cayenne pepper, seaweed flakes, cinnamon, turmeric, nama shoyu and Braggs Liquid Aminos.

People can ask for hemp, flax or other high omega three oil, which I did. Some people went in the sweet porridge direction with cinnamon as a sweetener and perhaps stevia too.

I formed a preference for a savoury version with cayenne pepper, turmeric, seaweed flakes and nama shoyu. This is still my breakfast most days and I did not stop there. I also chop up sunflower and snow pea greens and have them alongside, mixed with some of each of whatever sprouts I have growing at the time and some flax or hemp oil. I stir a pinch of cayenne and a teaspoonful of turmeric into the cooked quinoa or millet, drizzle it with oil and spray a little tamari over the top. In fact, it is a meal that could be enjoyed for lunch or dinner, but for breakfast I seem to be a creature of habit and make this countless times. I continue to enjoy it as much as ever and it sustains me through the morning.

....

A Full British Breakfast

Whether it is a full English, Scottish, or Welsh breakfast, this is fun to make on occasion, just because you can. It might be kinder to your system to wake up first with some green juice and then to have a full British as an early brunch.

Try some of these:

Aubergine or Courgette Rashers, marinated mushrooms, strips of red capsicum or sweet red pepper painted with oil and wilted in the dehydrator, **Sweet Potato-wrapped Chipolatas** (with or without the sweet potato wrapping) and **Red Pepper Ketchup.** Instead of baked beans, you could include sprouted red lentils in **Mild Red Pepper Sauce.** For a scramble, mix a little almond mayonnaise, grated courgettes, chopped avocado and a pinch of turmeric for the colour. For toast, serve dehydrated bread or crackers and **Butter Spread.**

Smoothies and Green Smoothies –

for breakfast or at other times

Smoothies are rapidly gaining popularity and bring a lot of good folk in the raw direction. The basic recipe is to put good things in a blender with water or juice and to make a thick milkshake-like creation, without the milk.

Green smoothies are usually blended from fresh greens, fruit, water, super food powders and perhaps ground seeds and nuts, such as hemp seeds.

Many are thankful for green smoothies as way of getting greens into people who do not like them. Smoothies mixing fruit and green vegetables present food combining challenges, but you can make vegetable and nut smoothies sweetened with stevia, and perhaps cinnamon. You can add in blue green algae, spirulina and chlorella powders, rice protein powder and whatever other food powders you are having. Try chard leaves, a carrot, algae powders, stevia and almonds. Smoothies need not be gourmet treats as long as they taste good enough to drink, but they should be sipped rather than gulped so that the body can sense them and start bringing the right enzymes towards them. Remember that every time you whip things up in blenders, oxidation takes place, so make sure you also chew plenty of raw vegetables during the day.

Greenshake

Smoothies are a good way of taking spirulina, chlorella and blue green algae and here is a recipe that tastes quite pleasant. It includes raw rice protein powder, see **Good Resources,** for easily assimilated protein and a factor that has been shown to be very helpful in healing from cancer.

Blend together these ingredients:

1 glass nut milk
½ small avocado
1 tablespoon raw rice protein powder
A few drops of vanilla extract
1 tablespoon in total of any of spirulina/chlorella/blue green algae
1 tiny spoon or drop of pure stevia extract
Small amounts of any other superfood powders that you are taking,
   such as a teaspoon of maca or slippery elm powder

Blended smoothies, green or otherwise, are not *drinks*, but blended foods. Juices can be rapidly absorbed into the blood stream, but smoothies contain blended fruit and/or vegetable fibre that has to be physically moved through the system by peristalsis. That puts smoothies in the same category as raw soups, raw sauces and well-chewed raw food. If you have too many meals, including smoothies, during the day it does not leave much recovery time for the gut lining and helpful gut bacteria colonies. Balance how many smoothies, snacks and meals you have in a day with consideration for digestive recovery time, your individual nutritional needs and the rhythm of your daily life.

Once you know smoothies are food, you can have one as a light breakfast, a snack or as part of a more substantial meal, and *also* have thirst-quenching drinks such as green juice, filtered water and herb tea in between. A smoothie on its own is not much of a meal at lunch or dinner and would probably not be sustaining enough. Of course fibre is very important, but there is plenty in raw vegetable meals, so in this way of eating fibre is not an issue.

This approach runs contrary to what some say about the benefits of having 'fibre-enriched' juices. Fibre in juices would be helpful if someone added green smoothies to a diet of mainly meat, refined flour and sugar products, but if you are eating plenty of sprouted foods and salad, shortage of fibre is not a problem.

Fruit smoothies make it too easy to eat a lot of fruit in a hurry, and that means a lot of sugar in one go. Instead, consider having a smaller amount of delicious ripe fruit as an occasional meal, chewed well.

....

Light Fruit Smoothie

Having said all this about fruit and sugar, people, including me sometimes, do love smoothies and they are lovely treats. I came up with this light fruit smoothie recipe. It is delicious and thick, but has far less sugar than regular smoothies. Per person, blend one piece of ripe organic fruit such as an unpeeled apple or peach, or a banana, with the juice of half a lemon and a cup of water. Sweeten to taste with pure stevia extract and thicken by blending in half an avocado. Add more water if you wish.

Savoury smoothies are on the same wavelength as raw soups. They are helpfully alkaline breakfasts and quick meals. Here is a fine recipe from fellow Hippocrates Health Educator, Jill Swyers:

Green Energy Soup Smoothie

1 tablespoon lemon juice	1 cup of sliced kale
4 tablespoons water	And/or:
2 cups chopped cucumber	1 cup Sunflower Greens
Half a lettuce	1 cup snowpea greens
1 clove of garlic, sliced	1 avocado
½ a mild onion, sliced	Mixed sprouts
3 sticks of celery, chopped	

Blend all the ingredients and season to taste with cayenne pepper, cumin, tamari, seaweed flakes…

Jill suggests adding more or less of each item according to your personal preference, which is pretty much how I prepare *all* my meals. It is a good way to make good smoothies, adding things until it is just right. As we get used to simple fresh food like this our tastes become more aligned with what is best for us at the time.

I think smoothies are good for:
- Meals in a hurry (but, to aid digestion, try to plan for relaxed mealtimes with time to sip and chew)
- Variety
- Making sure you eat enough very nourishing foods such as spirulina
- 'Survival rations' for work days and days out
- Snacks a long time away from your main meals
- Sneaking veggies into reluctant eaters
- When appetite is poor, and during illness, dentistry and convalescence
- The joy of smoothness

Good Drinks

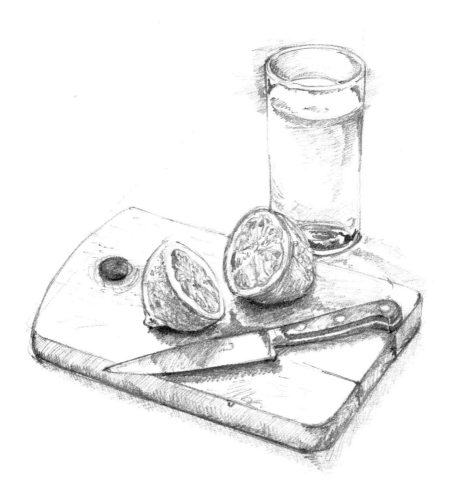

Lemonade

Hydration is as incredibly important, as we keep being told. All the miraculous activities of the cells need watery mediums. We take in water in raw vegetables, and then we need drinks between meals – between them rather than at them.

Drinks are better between meals, so that the digestive juices do not get washed away at meal times before engaging with the food.

Having said that, I would let a child drink when they are thirsty, whenever possible making sure they have plenty to drink a little while before the meal so that they are not thirsty when they sit down to eat.

Water

As well as watery drinks it is good to drink neat water. Spring water from a tested spring is ideal. If not that, what? Bottled water is fine, if it comes from a good source and is bottled in *glass*.

Avoid water from plastic bottles, unless that is all you can get when you are out. Plastic gives off chemicals which you really do not want to drink. Plastic bottles of water may have been warmed during transport, which would have let more chemicals leach into the water.

At home you might want to consider a filtration system. Jug filters help somewhat, and there are various options in between them and full house plumbed systems. A big problem these days is the quantities of pharmaceutical drugs that end up dissolved in the water, even after you filter it.

The option that removes pretty much everything you would not want is distilling water. Some do not like this way of getting pure water because it is too pure, without the minerals and subtle structures that water from a spring has. However, because of the pharmaceutical drug problem, perhaps you will want to investigate water systems for distilling water that work by by heating it and collecting the steam, or by collecting water from the atmosphere.

Meanwhile, at least get a filter jug and filter your tapwater. In the recipe ingredient lists I always say 'filtered water' as a reminder.

Do your homework and provide yourself with the cleanest freshest water you can find.

Lemon Juice

Ripe lemon juice squeezed into warm water is a good start to the day and a gently detoxing, alkalinising drink at any time.

....

Lemonade

Adding pure stevia extract powder or drops to lemon juice in water turns it into very good lemonade. I cannot detect any stevia aftertaste at all. Make it in big jugs for family life and for parties. Everyone I have given it to really likes it. I love stevia in my warm lemon juice in the morning.

....

Wheatgrass Juice

A juice, a drink, a supplement, an energy boost, a medicine, a magical elixir, whatever you call it, try giving wheatgrass juice a place in your daily life. Grow trays of wheatgrass at home, or buy them in, and have enough ready for a couple of ounces twice a day. You will be availing yourself of a drink that many, many people, including me, believe has vastly improved their wellbeing, and helped them to shrug off illness.

I found it challenging when I first started drinking wheatgrass, although others love it straight away. I had to sit down and look at a beautiful green plant, with a tasty raw cracker at my side. Next I would look at the beautiful green plant, think big thoughts about the rich plant life around the planet and swig down the juice. Then immediately I took the taste away by eating the cracker, and gave my stomach a different focus. After a week of this, morning and afternoon, I was able to manage the drink while looking at the plant and without the cracker. Now I find drinking wheatgrass juice no more pleasant or unpleasant than brushing my teeth.

Drink it neat, dilute it with water, or follow it with a chaser of water. Try holding it in your mouth and letting it start to digest. While you train yourself to like it, try lining up a glass of **lemonade** as a treat to drink afterwards. I am sure you will find a way that suits you.

Fresh wheatgrass juice is at its best in the first fifteen minutes from juicing. To make the most of your homegrown wheatgrass, pour a little filtered water into the fibre that comes from the juicer and put it back through the juicer. I am sure wheatgrass contributes to being and staying well, and to good energy levels, and that it is definitely worthwhile tending trays of growing grass.

If you do not have an auger juicer yet, you can blend your wheatgrass with filtered water and squeeze it through a mesh nut milk bag right into your glass.

••

Green Juice

Along with the wheatgrass juice, 'green juice' is foundational to the Hippocrates way of eating. Made in a good juicer that can squeeze out every last drop of nutritional juice, it adds so much to raw vegan living. It keeps energy levels up between meals and lessens or removes the need to snack. It can quell the taste for sweet snacks.

For me it seems to do that by meeting my nutritional needs. Then my system can stop hankering after quick sugar fixes and get on with the morning or afternoon's activities. When I have enough green juice I can easily avoid being attracted to sugary snacks. My energy levels stay higher and I do not find myself slumping with low energy or exhaustion. I have found it invaluable when unwell, and not hungry or ready for solid food.

For periods of fasting it is much safer and healthier than, for example, grape juice, carrot juice or water. I know people who have juice-fasted, or 'juice-feasted' on green juice for weeks, and who have felt the benefits while being able to carry on with normal life.

The basis for green juice is cucumber and celery, about ⅓ celery and ⅔ cucumber. If you can get it, use celery with all its leaves. For more nutrients including easily assimilable protein, it is important to add plenty of home grown or purchased tray-greens (snow pea, sunflower and buckwheat) and/or leafy greens. Depending on what is available locally and what you like, try spinach, chard, carrot leaves, stinging nettle leaves and other edible wild greens, dandelion leaves (if not too bitter for you), purple sprouting, broccoli leaves and stalks, kale, lettuce and green cabbage.

If you have a vegetable garden or allotment you will have plenty of green juice ingredients. Otherwise, frequent the nearest farmers' market and get green produce from as fresh and local a source as possible.

In spring and summer pick wild greens including young nettles and cleavers, if you know which plants to choose! These are as good as the extra-nourishing tray-grown greens.

Make sure you drink at least a litre of green juice a day. For the taste and the nutrition you can add garlic and or ginger to your juice. I love the ginger and hate the garlic, so it is very individual. You could see if adding lemon and/or stevia makes it easier to drink.

You can add blue green algae, preferably the defrosted fresh form, and spirulina and chlorella to your juices. I find I can stomach the defrosted fresh blue green algae in green juice but prefer the powdered forms in a **Greenshake** or in **Green Crisps.**

Green juice is not gourmet fare, but it can make such a difference to your life that it is worth getting over any initial discomfort at such an alkaline taste. Everyone I know who drinks green juice regularly says they come to like it, or at least finds drinking it a neutral experience. Try it for a month as an experiment, and you may not want to stop.

Before or for breakfast, mid-morning and mid-afternoon are the best times for drinking your green juice. Take it with you when you go out to keep your energy levels up without the succumbing to the temptations of the commercial snack market.

Ideally, make the juice freshly each time. That is not an ideal I live up to because I have other things to do in my day. I juice enough for the whole day, drink some, put the rest in a glass bottle, and keep it in the fridge. If I were seriously ill I would want to have fresh juice each time.

....

Green Water

The fibres from making green juice still have some green life in them. What I do is to add filtered water to the container of fibres and spoon it back through the juicer. The result is not a concentrated juice, but a green water that has some good nutrition in it. I have that instead of water now and then during the day and sometimes (depending on what greens I used) use it in savoury recipes as a stock instead of water.

....

Herb Tea

Mint, chamomile, lemon grass, ginger, liquorice... we are spoilt for choice for herb teas these days, and we can be cheated. You *must* read the small print because many mixed herb teas contain flavourings. The fruit teas can be the worst culprits. They say 'natural flavourings' but those flavourings are likely to be chemically extracted and may be nature-identical compounds and not the named plant at all! This is a pity because people may think they are buying something healthy when they are buying the unknown and probably untested.

Herb tea should be a step up from caffeinated drinks. My choice is to stick to simple herb teas, such as mint, when I am out, and to read the ingredient lists carefully before choosing packets to take home. If it says 'natural flavours', do not buy it.

Real herb teas edge into herbal medicine and can be very beneficial. Remember the joys of fresh herb teas too, and try teas made from mint, sage, rosemary and whatever herbs you have growing in your garden. Pick wild herbs and berries for tea, if you know what you are doing. Elderberries, rosehips and hawthorn berries together make very good 'fruit tea'. Elderflowers, European lime tree blossom and hawthorn flowers are delicately delightful.

....

Fruit juice

I avoid it, except for a rare treat from a juice bar when out. It has far too much sugar in it. By the time you have drunk the juice of a chunk of pineapple, a few oranges and a couple of apples (a typical juice-bar juice) you have drunk a lot of sugar. If fruit is not ripe it will draw from your body's resources to create balance. That is quite an issue considering the amount of fruit there is in a fruit juice.

Fruit juice is acid-forming in the system, which can undo your efforts at establishing a better alkaline/acid balance in your body. It was strange, after years of buying cartons, to find my tastes have changed and I really do not miss fruit juice. Even if I did, I would rather have steady energy from drinking green juice than the 'up followed by slump' I get from too much sugar, in fruit or in any other form. That is why I do not put carrots in my green juice. Carrot tops yes, carrots no, too acid-forming. However, when you are getting used to green juice you could add some carrot or fruit to make it palatable so that you can at least get into a green juice habit.

Light Fruit Juice

But fruit juice is very pleasant, and when you make it yourself it is a fresher more healthful beverage than commercially packaged juice. Here is my recipe for a lighter version, sweetened with stevia. Make it in jugs for a party treat. Per serving, juice one piece of ripe organic fruit such as an apple, pear or peach, or the equivalent of grapes, berries or other fruit. Mix with 1½ cups filtered water or more, the juice of half a lemon and a little pure stevia extract to taste. You might not want lemon juice with more tart berries such as black currants. This proportion of fruit gives a delicious fruit taste and is more thirst-quenching than regular juice.

....

Carrot Juice

I use carrot juice and carrots in recipes, but it is too sweet to drink in whole glasses. Having said that, do put some carrot juice in your green juice, just for a while, if it helps you get used to the green vegetable tastes. Carrots have many good qualities, but when you put them in salads and other recipes the quantity per serving is far less.

....

Almond Milk

Almond milk is delicious and nutritious, and very easy to make. It is a good protein drink for building up strength. Try making this quantity at first, doubling the recipe if you wish once you are used to it. You will need a nut milk bag from a raw food site online or a jelly-making bag from a cook shop, which are basically the same thing, fine mesh bags.

1 cup almonds
2 cups filtered water, plus a further two or more cups to dilute the
  milk if you wish

Soak the almonds overnight or all day. If you want to use the fibres for another recipe, rub the skins off so that the fibres will be white and less coarse.

If you are just making the milk this does not matter. Blend the almonds and water until as smooth as possible.

Arrange the mesh bag over a large bowl. Pour the blended mixture into the bag and squeeze the milk through into the bowl. If you will be using the fibres in a different recipe, do not bother to squeeze out every drop of milk because a little will be good with the fibres.

Use this rich creamy milk as it is in recipes such as **Almond Milk Mayonnaise**.

For drinking, dilute with two, or more to taste, further cups of water, putting the water back through the fibres to get the most milk out of them. Flavour to taste with any of these: pure stevia extract, cinnamon, ginger and vanilla. Warm it for a nourishing bedtime drink by warming over the lowest heat while stirring with your clean finger. Try adding a teaspoon of soothing slippery elm powder or hormone-balancing maca.

Nut Milk Varieties

Following the almond milk recipe, you can make milk with various nuts and seeds (except flax/linseed and chia/Mila which would swell up and make a jelly). Try hemp seeds, sesame seeds and hazelnuts.

If you use hemp seeds with their hulls removed you can simply blend them up with water, using more or less filtered water according to how rich and concentrated you want the milk to be. With their hulls, make hemp milk in the same way as almond milk.

Super Nut Milk
(Protein-rich)

Pollen is well worth keeping around as a helpful 'superfood'. The pollen adds sweetness to the creaminess of the milk. This is a nourishing drink to take out with you as a liquid snack, a good 'transition food' to help in your worthy efforts to stay away from junk snacks.

Add a tablespoon of pollen to a glass of nut milk. Leave for a while for the pollen to soak and dissolve in the milk. Add any of these to taste: a tiny spoon or drop of pure stevia extract, a pinch of cinnamon or ginger powder, a few drops of vanilla extract. If you take any other superfood powders you could add them as well. Try a teaspoon of maca or chlorella.

....

Rice Protein Powder Shakes

There are various protein shake powders on the market, especially in the fitness market, and the best of all so far seem to be made from raw, sprouted rice. See **Good Resources**. These are good for increasing your protein intake for wellbeing, recovery and muscle development. They also taste great.

I take the vanilla one, enjoying it stirred up as a milkshake or warm drink so that it is a treat. It is sweetened with stevia. It is good mixed with home made almond milk and is a helpful drink to take out with you. I imagine it has some fibre, but nowhere near as much as a regular smoothie. You can mix it with spirulina, chlorella and bluegreen algae for a sweet green shake.

Slippery Elm Malted Milk

Slippery elm is a mild-tasting powder from the bark of the slippery elm tree, slippery-textured when mixed with water. I mean plain slippery elm powder, not 'Slippery elm food' that is slippery elm mixed with wheat flour and other things that you might not want.

Slippery elm has the reputation of being healing and soothing to the intestinal lining. Try mixing a spoonful with warm oat or almond milk and perhaps a tiny spoon or drop of pure stevia extract, as an evening drink. It has a faintly malted taste.

··

Coffee Substitutes

You can buy quite a few different coffee substitutes made from roasted grains, chicory or dandelions. Some are processed so that they are instant and some are ground so that you can use them like ground coffee. It is not wonderful nutrition, but it might help you to stop drinking coffee.

Hot Carob

Carob not only has a good rich taste similar to chocolate, but it is sweet. For a rich thick drink, stir a spoonful in almond or oat milk and warm it in a pan by stirring with a clean finger over a low heat. It is comforting, nourishing and tastes very good.

Steamed Soymilk

I do not touch soymilk as a rule. Soya products are not easy to digest, except for the traditional fermented ones – miso, tamari/nama shoyu and tempeh. There are serious questions about how unfermented soya affects our natural hormone balances. However, when stranded far from home in a chain coffee shop, it is occasionally good to have something other than more mint tea. If a steamed soymilk can keep you off coffee, so be it. Try it with cinnamon and nutmeg. Some more awake cafés now offer oat or rice milk, so things are looking up.

Social Drinking

What about times when the others are drinking wine, beer and other alcoholic drinks? Once you understand that alcohol creates a sugar problem in the body as well as being quite toxic (and, ironically, dehydrating) you might be happy to give it up, or at least to cut back.

Sparkling mineral water looks festive and makes a change, however it is acidic, so not good as a daily choice. If you usually avoid it, a glass of fruit juice, perhaps diluted with mineral water, so that it lasts you longer and has less of a concentration of sugar, can become a treat.

Of the fruit juices, grapefruit is the least sweet. I like it ½ and ½ with mineral water. Some people find it is the social pressure to drink alcoholic drinks that is the problem, not resisting the alcohol itself. If that is so, find a coach like me, someone with NLP skills or similar, who can help you to reframe how you respond in situations where drinking alcohol is the norm. That kind of support can also help you get beyond food addictions.

Why Water?

Our bodies have a large proportion of water, an inner ocean. It is the medium for all the activity in the body, the all-important electrical activity and transport of nutrients and wastes. Blood, lymph, movement, thinking, healing, growing, imagining, detoxing, coping with change, all require plenty of water. That is why I make such a fuss about it in a recipe book.

By drinking plenty of good water between meals, whether filtered, distilled or from a spring, you will make the best use of all the good food that you are creating and eating. *Santé!* Cheers!

How To Invent Raw Dishes

This is what you can do:

Read my raw recipes and other people's, and start changing them. Chop some olives into the paté. Crunch up some dehydrated raw corn chips and use them as a garnish. Try a different combination of vegetables in the salad. Spread leftover raw dips on non-stick baking sheets and see what happens when you dehydrate them. Look at the salad sections of regular recipe books and get ideas from the pictures.

If you enjoy some cooked food, start wondering what you might make that would be similar, only with no cooking. Some of my recipes originated that way. Some I figured out from memories.

Think hard about cooked foods you like. What is it about them? Texture? Flavours? How could you get that in a different way? My raw oatcakes are an example. I was buying regular oatcakes to top up my raw food and decided to go one better. What are your favourites that you would still like to enjoy, and how can you create something with similar textures and tastes?

Take risks and try new fusions of cultural flavours. Tacos with Thai fillings? Seaweed nori rolls with Italian herbs and avocado? Dishes that honour your own cultural roots in new ways?

Make mistakes. My raw Haggis was the worst raw dish I ever made. I will not give out a raw vegan Haggis recipe until I figure out a delicious one. Do not let a spectacular failure stop you. If you do not like something you make, add other ingredients or change it into something quite different.

Inventing no-cook dishes is much easier than inventing cooked ones because you do not have to worry about oven temperatures and cooking times. What you prepare is pretty much what you will get – except with dehydrated creations. Under-season those because the flavours become more concentrated as the water dries out.

What Is Behind
This Way Of Eating?

The Hippocrates Way

Raw and living food is not a strict diet and need not be dull, restrictive or weird. The *New York Times* called it 'The most important diet in the 21st century'.

I call it the Hippocrates Way because I learned it at the Hippocrates Health Institute, where it has been the way that in 50 years has helped many thousands of people heal and vastly improve the quality of their lives.

By contrast, some prescriptive diets from the teaching of a single expert, and some raw food diets, may be unbalanced and less likely to achieve those results. Magazines and papers write about those diets and they are often fads. A particular diet may be an improvement on what someone was eating before and might work for a while, but it may not be balanced enough for long-term wellbeing.

The Hippocrates Health Institute is a world-class spa and education centre in Florida that was rated the world's number one teaching institute in 2000 by Spa Management Group. It is a thriving and evolving centre that was founded by visionary humanitarian raw and living food pioneers, Ann Wigmore and Viktoras Kulvinskas, and is currently under the leadership of Dr Brian and Dr Anna Maria Clement.

Dr Brian Clement, a clear-thinking and visionary scientist with remarkable vitality, travels the world teaching people this way of eating. Consider going to one of his talks around the world, and watch him on Youtube. He can deservedly take a bow for the applause from countless people whose lives he has helped to transform, and even save.

Many people who go to the Hippocrates Health Institute (or learn from Hippocrates Health Educators, like me, who teach these guidelines) after mainstream medical services have given up on them have become well again, and able to get on with their lives. Diagnosis can become a signal for some extra work rather than an indication of a dire, and possibly short, life sentence.

At The Hippocrates Heath Institute life follows tried and tested guidelines for aiding healing from life-threatening illness and lesser ailments, and for optimum wellbeing. Evidence comes from over 30 years of clinical experience and research, and from the life stories of the thousands of people who have stayed there and transformed their lives.

The Hippocrates way differs from the approaches of many in raw food circles. In mainstream cultures around the world the focus tends to be on the sensory quality of food. Not surprisingly, many transfer this focus to raw vegan food and create meals by combining whatever raw ingredients taste good together – without working with the science and results of research that point to what works best for wellness.

That popular approach to raw food provides big steps forward from what most people eat. It can be a sensible rule of thumb, and one that allows intuition to play its part in making food choices. There is freedom and simplicity in taking on 100% raw as a rule, and then working from any raw food recipes. There are plenty of popular approach raw recipe books and recipes available online now. When making a move into raw food, for some people that may be a good way forward. Some teachers with that kind of approach know a great deal and have much to teach.

In fact, there is so much invention in raw food that in future it will develop far beyond the current repertoires of growing numbers of raw chefs and recipe creators who are contributing to this relatively new cuisine. I am grateful for their inspiration.

However, the lack of consensus in raw food circles has been confusing for people looking to make the best raw vegan food choices for wellbeing. This is important to notice, since the range of people wanting to make the best choices includes everyone from young top athletes to people of all ages trying to recover quickly from catastrophic illness. To address this, some of the most experienced and knowledgeable leading raw food teachers meet together for 'Raw Food Summits', at which optimum diet standards were agreed. For more depth, look in **Good Resources** for Diana Store's book *Raw Food Works* with contributions by these experts. I met some of them when they were holding a summit the second time I stayed at the Hippocrates Health Institute. They were sincere, thoughtful, fascinating and knowledgeable people with a vast amount of long term practical experience with raw and living food. The Hippocrates way lies within their guidelines.

On the Hippocrates way you stride into territory in which you can have *both* delicious satisfying food *and* optimal nutrition for wellness. To me it feels right intuitively, as well as logically.

You do not have to take this way on, or to take it on all at once (although you can), but these recipes can sustain and delight you while contributing to your healing. I hope they will put a spring in *your* step, as they have in mine.

Follow the Hippocrates guidelines for

- ✿ Vastly improving your energy and fitness levels
- ✿ Detoxing and re-establishing optimum health
- ✿ An established pathway with a first class success rate
- ✿ A balanced diet with scientific backing
- ✿ Helping yourself or a member of your household through serious illness
- ✿ Giving your digestive system an easy time
- ✿ Avoiding and easily recovering from common ailments
- ✿ A complete balanced vegan diet
- ✿ Ageing gracefully – and only slowly!
- ✿ Food to support clear thinking and spiritual/emotional development
- ✿ Sustenance for carrying out your life plans

My Version of the Hippocrates Way of Eating

After nine weeks eating, studying, and getting fit as a flea, at the Hippocrates Health Institute in Florida, I returned to cold Edinburgh weather. I had to break my 'rules' when caught out without sufficient ideal nourishing foods. It was better to eat cooked food than to go hungry and feel cold. I had Scottish oatcakes, hot curries, Thai and other cooked vegetarian food (as well as plenty of good raw food and juices). Many of my dehydrator recipes come from creating better satisfying, healthy alternatives and pocket snacks.

As a naturally thin person I need to eat a lot to keep up my weight, keep well, and to keep warm when it is cold. The Hippocrates **Green Juice** for breakfast would not be enough for my thin self, and in Florida I gratefully ate bowls of cooked millet and quinoa in the mornings. At home I evolved a breakfast with cooked millet or quinoa, condiments from the Hippocrates buffet choices and chopped tray greens and sprouts, eaten quite soon after my morning green drink. See **A Favourite Breakfast.** It is in the breakfast recipe section, but would be a good meal at any time if you eat some cooked food. I never tire of it, and my visitors ask for it.

Almost without fail I have the three **Green Juice** drinks, or more, a day and, honestly, I quickly grew to love them. I find it impossible to grow enough tray greens for half my green juice, but I add what I can, and also plenty of nourishing green vegetables including wild greens.

My juices include some of these: carrot tops, stinging nettles, chard, beet tops, kale and other greens, as well as two or three cucumbers to a head of celery. When I can, I get celery with its green leaves attached. I take bottles of green juice out with me and often add spirulina, chlorella and blue green algae powders so that it is a very sustaining drink. It moves my focus away from pointless money-wasting junk snacks.

For treats and when the occasion offered no good alternatives I have eaten all sorts of stuff. As a gourmet-type who plays with tastes and textures in my own creations, I seriously like variety and gourmet treats. Meat I easily refuse, but saying 'no' to cheese boards, good chocolate and an occasional proper French pastry is hard.

But, I know what I can get away with. I feel the effects of these things in my system and they are rare exceptions to my habits. I cannot indulge myself at every opportunity because there are far too many opportunities! This was difficult at first, especially with chocolate, and I have had phases when it became difficult again. What finally made the difference was personal development work to change unhelpful old beliefs. I share this work with people in my coaching and consultancy because it makes this way of eating very easy.

Anyone seriously ill should stick to the Hippocrates way. It is the 'gold standard'. I indulge in unhelpful foods less and less because I enjoy being well so much.

At home I:
- ☘ grow wheatgrass, sprouts and tray greens
- ☘ drink two ounce wheatgrass shots twice a day (or once fresh and once powdered)
- ☘ drink green juice three times a day
- ☘ eat according to the guidelines and recipes in this book

I would not trust living on mainly raw foods without the wheatgrass, green juices, sprouted foods, tray greens, seaweeds, algae and other good ingredients that you will find here. I believe knowing all this is far more important than indiscriminately eating 100% raw vegan food.

A Good Daily Rhythm

This is the basic rhythm of life at the Hippocrates Health Institute. I have been following it when possible since the beginning of 2008. Here is a daily rhythm that you can work with.

On waking: Fresh lemon juice in a large glass of filtered water, perhaps with sweet pure stevia extract. The alkalising lemon juice helps to continue the night's natural detox. The water is rehydrating, which wakes you up and cleans your oesophagus.

Soon after waking: Approximately 2 ounces or 50ml freshly prepared **Wheat Grass Juice.** This is both highly nutritious and helpfully detoxing. It gives a tremendous boost of energy, without taxing the nervous system as tea or coffee would.

Around 9:00, or before going to work: A large glass of **Green Juice**. In this basic rhythm the first green juice of the day serves as breakfast and that may be enough. Some have people have fruit, perhaps three days a week, and some have a bowl of cooked quinoa or millet (See the **Good Breakfasts** section for further possibilities).

Mid-morning: Green Juice

Lunch: Main meal of sprouts, vegetable salads, and either protein rich or carbohydrate rich choices.

Late afternoon: Third drink of **Green Juice.**

Between green juice and dinner: Second drink of 2oz/50ml of freshly prepared **Wheatgrass Juice**

Dinner: As lunch, perhaps slightly lighter. If lunch was a carbohydrate rich meal perhaps dinner can be a protein rich meal. This does not matter, as long as you have some of each over time. This way of eating really does provide plenty of protein and it is perfectly OK to simply finish up what you made for lunch for dinner. You will not go short of protein.

Drinks: Filtered water, and lemon, herb teas and occasional coffee substitute drinks. See the **Good Drinks** chapter for further suggestions.

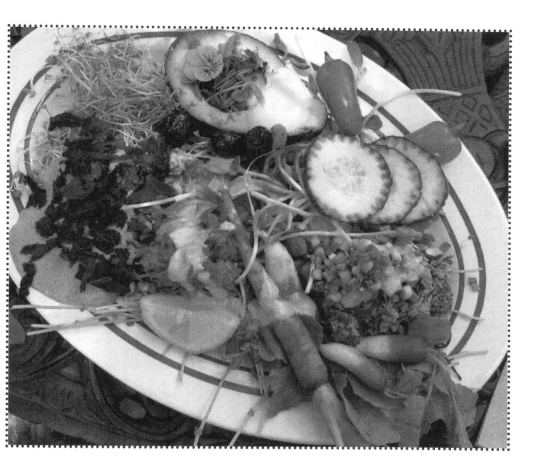

A plate of food from the Hippocrates Health Institute
Lunch Buffet

Warmth

If you live in a warm climate warm food may be optional, but if you live somewhere cold it is a necessity.

The Hippocrates buffet in Florida may make your mouth water and provides a perfect array of colours, flavours and textures, but try facing a salad when arriving home cold in a British December, and waiting for the central heating to warm the place up. You would have to be 'staunch' to crunch into cold salad from the fridge unless you are already feeling warm, and I am not sure how wise it would be.

Many nutritional and healing systems stress the importance of hot foods. How can that be squared with the Hippocrates way? Chinese medicine, for example, stresses the importance of warmth, particularly to support healing specific health conditions. Rudolf Steiner spoke of the importance of warmth in food.

Raw foods have rich available nutrition with intact enzymes, but there is no law about eating them stone cold! Here are some suggestions for warming things up:

- Blend up a raw soup from the **Good Soups** chapter and warm it over the lowest heat, either stirring with your finger or keeping the temperature below 115° Fahrenheit/46° centigrade with a thermometer
- Have steamed vegetables such as leeks, sweet potatoes and broccoli with cold pressed olive oil and tamari or a gently warmed raw sauce, and a sprout salad. By the time you have eaten some hot vegetables you might relish the salad – especially with the **Hippocrates House Dressing**, which I find appetising even on cold days
- Use cayenne pepper, as a sprinkle in tiny quantities, in sauces and as an ingredient in savouries, for a different kind of warmth
- Make well-spiced raw Asian dishes with cayenne pepper
- Serve some hot grain-like seed, such as quinoa, along with raw dishes
- Make cooked vegan soup or stew and count it in your 20% cooked food

✿ Eat oats to warm your system. Have soaked raw oats for breakfast and try my dehydrated **Oat Cakes**

These suggestions may help you to stay warm. Also remember to wear enough warm clothes! Many people do not, but if you keep your inner fires banked up with warm layers of clothing then warmth from food is less of an issue.

Good Cooked Food

At the Hippocrates Health Institute people fill their plates from delicious raw buffets. They also serve simple vegetable and lentil soups sometimes, and cooked millet and quinoa and steamed vegetables are available for those who need them. Organic sprouted grain breads are sometimes offered as wraps for salad dishes.

Dr Brian Clement, Dr Anna Maria Clement and the other top health practitioners and experts who meet for the 'Raw Food Summits' have found that when at least 80% of someone's food is organic, raw and living, and they eat an overall healthy alkaline balance of organic vegan ingredients, *and they are already well,* then the same level of wellness can be maintained on 80% raw as on 100% raw food.

What are some good cooked food choices?
✿ Steamed vegetables
✿ Steamed/boiled millet, quinoa and buckwheat, preferably soaked and rinsed first
✿ Vegan curries, casseroles and soups (made at home without browning the vegetables)

Less good, but still better than most standard food, are:
✿ Occasional *air*-popped corn – *not* oil-popped corn and *not* microwave-popped – corn (*not* microwaved *anything*)
✿ Wheat-free bread and pasta made from rye, rice and corn
✿ Soft corn tortillas

- ♣ Oat porridge
- ♣ Oat cakes
- ♣ Vegan curries, casseroles and soups when eating out

Avoid grilled, roasted and fried foods, so that you do not get the damaged fats and oils and deeply browned or burnt food surfaces that are carcinogenic (cancer-causing). This rules out barbecues, sorry. For cooked food when camping and eating in nature, wrap sweet potatoes in foil and bake them in the embers, or boil things up.

The best methods for cooking are steaming, boiling, and occasionally gently baking vegetables without burning them. Instead of grilling and oven-cooking get really good results similar to cooked tastes and textures by marinating food and using a dehydrator.

If you choose to have up to 20% cooked food you can come up with interesting raw/cooked combinations. Thinking this way is helpful when making a transition into eating more raw food. Try these:

- ♣ A raw curry with both steamed millet and grated courgette 'rice', and raw chutney
- ♣ Cooked lentils in a raw soup
- ♣ Dehydrated raw vegan burgers or sausages with mashed steamed sweet potatoes, raw gravy and a sprout salad
- ♣ Raw sauces over steamed vegetables
- ♣ Asian-style mixtures of finely chopped raw vegetables, spices and seasonings (perhaps marinated and or lightly dehydrated) mixed with cooked millet or, occasionally, cooked brown rice

Very occasionally for special meals, I *lightly* fry good corn tortillas, and offer raw Mexican-type fillings including guacamole, sprouts, salsas, nut cream and finely sliced salad ingredients. Much better though are dehydrated raw **Corn Tortillas**.

Just as rarely, I make buckwheat pancakes from a batter of blended, sprouted buckwheat. I take care not to over-brown them and discard burnt ones. These are definitely *not* the best of cooked foods, but are so much better than what is out there in the 'real' world in, for example, infamous hamburger chains. Worst of all has to be the Scottish 'delicacy' of the deep fried Mars Bar! People actually eat them. They contribute nothing to wellness.

It is not just for wellness that I eat raw food. I really like it! There is so much flavour and vitality in it. My *tastes* keep changing even further towards simple, fresh and raw. When I have cooked food, however much I enjoy it, I start yearning for raw food and, quite naturally and quickly, I get back to raw food and find it more satisfying. I know I can eat plenty, have energy for digestion, and have plenty of energy for happy busy days.

Raw food is much better emotionally. With wellbeing comes lightness, steadiness and happier emotions.

Add to that clearer and brighter thought processes, mental and physical agility, strength and stamina, and it is obvious why I continue on this way of eating, and why I recommend it to you wholeheartedly.

Sunshine and Food

Life on earth depends on sunshine. Carnivore and herbivore animals, green plants and sea plants, fungi, bacteria and viruses, all exist in a long interdependent web of being that depends on the sun.

Rudolf Steiner spoke about sunshine and food. In a sense, when you eat green food you eat the sunshine involved in photosynthesis. If you eat meat from animals that ate the green food they get the sunshine, and you do not. Even if at first it sounds far fetched, it is worth meditating on sunshine and food.

When green food is cooked, the cell walls get broken and the food is easier to digest, but now we have juicers and blenders we do not have to rely on cooking to save us all the chewing. Rather than literally cooking the living daylights out of all our food we can enjoy most or all of it raw.

Other People

Children

Children who play in the kitchen learn how to feed themselves for life. When they are involved in chopping, sprouting, blending, growing, juicing and decorating they are so open to eating and enjoying the food.

Making food is enjoyable playtime. Let them stamp out carrot stars, make date marzipan shapes, cut up vegetables, roll up wraps, blend their own smoothies, turn the handle to make raw vegetable pasta and spread out cracker mixtures on dehydrator sheets. Decorate patés and create fantasy cakes for and with them. Pick edible flowers together and let them arrange them on the food.

Pick wild food together and teach them the names of the plants as you learn them. This can go on for years, and then they will effortlessly know how prepare good meals when they are older.

As you find your way you can introduce more raw food to your children. With teenagers it can be different and you may need to go easy. My daughter, who was brought up on mainly vegan food with sprouts and a lot of salads, had this to say:

> 'When I was 16 I basically only wanted to eat normal things like white pasta and cheese. Slowly I worked out what made my body feel better and began to mind less what my friends thought, and now my friends think I am pretty cool. At 16 I did not want to drink green juice in the morning and eat sprouts for breakfast, although I frequently do now. I certainly learned a lot from my mother, but I had to discover these things for myself and to learn from people other than her as well. Initially, resisting these things was part of that journey.'

Couples

Everything depends on how compatible your tastes and eating habits are. Open-minded people can usually find a way forward. Can you prepare the food that is right for you while they prepare other food? Emma MacDoughall explores couple dynamics in *Me Raw You Cooked* (see **Good Resources).**

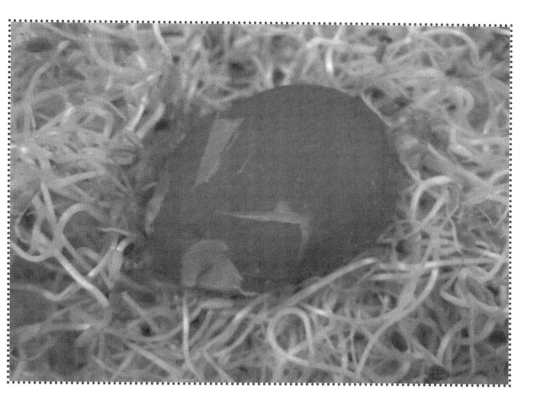

A Happy Radish Mouse Eating a Nest of Sprouts

Families and Gatherings

When people eat together meals can be buffets with a variety of dishes on offer. Each person takes what suits them. I know raw folk who provide only raw food for visitors. I usually do, but it depends on their needs. When visitors and family are around I usually play and experiment with raw dishes, but sometimes offer cooked vegetables, grains, and occasionally eggs or goats cheese. People are grateful for exquisite good food and usually do not care that it is vegan and raw. They are usually fascinated by it.

A Household of One

In a raw household of one you can fill your fridge and cupboards with just what suits you, and generally please yourself.

Here are some tips from my experience:

- ⚜ Make two platefuls of dinner. Put one in the fridge or in your lunch box. Later it feels as if mum provided your meal!
- ⚜ Buy dried herbs and spices in small quantities so they get used while still fresh
- ⚜ Try not to over-buy produce. Then you can see to the back of the fridge, and are not trying to catch up with yourself
- ⚜ Make dips, spreads, salsas, dressings, pestos, and pâtés in small quantities to use while they are still fresh
- ⚜ Get just as good quality equipment as for a larger household
- ⚜ Get a small blender like the Tribest Blender that comes with extra containers and lids for carrying food and drinks
- ⚜ Get a nine-tray dehydrator so you can make plenty of food at one time, and then store in airtight containers

The Wider World

If raw is working for you, brilliant. Your face might be radiating and you might be beaming energy in all directions. When we are excited and learning new things we want to share and talk about them. Not everyone is ready to learn these things at the same time. They may even react negatively, and feel judged for eating their steak and kidney pie as you serve up your delicious 'courgetti' and get enthusiastic about living enzymes.

Reaching out to the wider raw food community at potlucks and talks, and online, is a good way to air your experiences and to share your challenges and triumphs with people who are equally excited and who are also experimenting with raw food.

My daughter says:

> *'When I bring sprouts and pots of my mum's dehydrated kale crisps to work my teenage students are curious and want to try them. They like them and want to learn more. This is because they have seen what I do and are interested in the way I live.'*

Meet the people in your life where they are, with acceptance, patience and empathy. Spark curiosity. Invite them to taste morsels of your delicacies. First and foremost, enjoy your own wellness journey.

Eating from a Corner Shop

There are times for doing your best with what is available. Here are four bright ideas for using what you can find in the nearest shop:

- **Bought hummus and cucumber**. Buy a pot of hummus and a cucumber. Wash the cucumber if you are near a sink, snap it in half and dip it in the hummus. That is the lunch snack you can find almost anywhere.
- **Bought soup with chopped leaves**. Buy a carton of good quality vegetable soup and a bag of 'designer salad leaves'. While you are gently warming the soup in your friend's home, chop all the leaves very finely, the finer the better. Serve the soup, allowing it to cool slightly if you brought it to a boil. Sprinkle the chopped leaves on the top and enjoy. Try Spicy lentil soup and chopped watercress, or carrot and coriander soup with chopped mixed leaves including herbs. Any bag of greens will be delicious.
- **Rice crackers and avocado.** Spreading ripe avocado on rice crackers makes an easy lunch, even though there is little food value in rice cakes. Or, just eat the avocado.

- ♣ **A box of salad and a packet of nuts.** Buy a box of mixed salad and sprinkle a packet of nuts, preferably not roasted, on the top. You could squeeze some lemon juice over the salad instead of opening the dressing sachet.

What To Eat When Out and at Functions and Conferences

Here are some good possibilities:
- ♣ Choose several different side salads, or a plate of salad and a side dish of steamed vegetables, instead of a main meal
- ♣ Take some **Salad Dressing Flakes** and sprinkle them over plain salad
- ♣ Book ahead and ask for raw vegan food
- ♣ Have a vegetarian curry or similar, and ask for green salad instead of rice
- ♣ Ask for salad with your soup instead of the bread
- ♣ Find somewhere with a salad bar or buffet
- ♣ For better food combining, choose a starter and a main instead of a main and a dessert.

Where to Eat Out

- ♣ Raw cafes and restaurants. Hooray! More of these are springing up. They may be expensive and good food combinations may not feature on the menu, but they are great for special occasions, and for inspiration.
- ♣ Anywhere that serves big fresh salads. Ask for oil and lemon to dress your salad instead of having their acidic regular vinegar dressing. Or take along **Salad Dressing Flakes**
- ♣ Salad bars where you get to pick and choose
- ♣ Vegetarian restaurants – though some may serve rather heavy food
- ♣ Indian, especially vegetarian Southern Indian, and Thai restaurants. They do delicious vegan/vegetarian food. Quite often they do interesting salads or combined cooked/salad dishes, with no wheat. Ask them for some green salad instead of the rice.

- ❧ Chinese restaurants that will leave out the MSG for you
- ❧ Mexican restaurants, sticking to the salads, beans and corn tortilla/rice-based dishes
- ❧ Juice bars. These tend to serve blended fresh or frozen fruits, and perhaps fruit/vegetable mixtures. You risk a sugar-rush. The fancy names are hype. When I have asked, people have been happy to juice or blend different combinations of fruits for me, or just vegetables if they have them. I have a juice bar juice or smoothie occasionally if it feels right, but not with other food. I rejoice and pay up when I spot wheatgrass shots in airports and on big stations. That *really* is a boost.

East, West, Home is Best

Other than going to the Hippocrates Health Institute or the Tree of Life Rejuvenation Centre (see **Good Resources**) and having your food and juice prepared for you, the best food for wellness will be the food you prepare at home, day after day. I hope these recipes make it much easier for you to prepare just the right meals. Often big salads with plenty of sprouts and a delicious dressing may be enough. Some days you may want to get busy in the kitchen and to follow the more involved recipes.

If you have a dehydrator, have a 'baking' day at home sometimes, making a few different things. Then you will have dried food to store for making easy meals on busy days. With so many interesting ingredients and ways of preparing foods available to you, I am sure you will be delighted with your creations.

Enjoy the food, enjoy wellbeing, enjoy plenty of energy and enjoy your life.

My Food Story

In South African sunshine I was weaned on mashed avocados and ripe fruit.

I grew up in England on the vegetables my father grew. We ate beautifully cooked plain meat and vegetable meals, and freshly picked salad in season. We had local meat, jersey milk and brown bread, 'the fat of the land', all pretty much organic, although it was not called that then.

My mother, a biologist and chemist, read nutrition books by Gayelord Hauser and Adele Davies. She gave us vitamin C tablets, and hot lemon and honey for colds. She encouraged my love of nature and I roamed the woods exploring, playing and eating blackberries, elderberries, strawberries, hawthorn leaves, beach leaves, Beach nuts, sorrel, hazelnuts and dandelions. Fruits were collected for pies and jam, elderflowers for syrup and champagne, cowslips for wine, and nettles and sorrel for soup. All my childhood I played in the kitchen. I still do.

I grew up with a strong connection to the earth and to food, along with a knowledge of botany and nutrition. At school I embarked on A level Biology. It was half OK dissecting a dogfish. I liked my neat little dissecting kit, but there was no way I would dissect a rabbit. It was too much like a wild creature, or my cat, and should not have died for me. I fled the laboratory and sat in tears weighing up my academic future and my conscience. My conscience won, but I needed another A Level.

Days later my kind Head Mistress made me an offer too perfect, exciting and miraculous to refuse. They were planning a Cookery A Level course for the following year. The teacher would teach just me while preparing for the bigger group. After refusing to cut up a rabbit I became a guinea pig!

Imagine a third of your timetable for two years with your own wonderful cookery teacher/fellow food enthusiast! Soon there was nothing I could not cook. I loved it.

After A levels I was an au pair in Paris, cooking French food for seven and eating in the best restaurants. I bought *Larousse Gastronomique* in English, for all the recipes since the court chefs set up restaurants and delicatessens after the French revolution.

Imagine me next as a student in Brighton, living on full English breakfasts in a drafty seaside hotel, and eating chips, macaroni cheese, bread, pies, custard and trifle in the college canteen. South coast winds whipped through me. Perhaps sugar, wheat, dairy and the weather caused my sore throats. Goodbye dear tonsils.

I gained weight. I was not fat but I did not feel good. I bought special vitamin toffees that were supposed to stop me feeling hungry. They did not. I just binged on them when I was writing essays, and ate all the food as well.

When I moved into a flat, things improved. People liked my meals, a lot. I went to a vegetarian café and ate strange new dishes, including one with soaked wheat berries. Infinity Foods opened in Brighton with bins of dried ingredients to scoop into paper bags. This was a new way. We ate every combination of rice, lentils, beans, vegetables, nuts and seeds. Sprouts appeared in little jars on our kitchen windowsill.

After university we had plans to open a vegetarian restaurant in Oxford. The finances fell through, but it would have been ahead of its time, and good. 'Love and Peas' was a possible name and 'Jam, Juicy and Jelly' from our names – Janet, Judy and Jenny, was another.

I learned from travelling. World cuisine, yes! Malaysia, Singapore and Indonesia; eating in cafes and from street stalls. Bliss. Italy, Greece, Yugoslavia, Turkey, Iran and Afghanistan, eating all the way. I discovered coriander leaves piled high on cloths on the pavement in Iran and sprinkled sour ground sumac berries over my rice. I discovered tempeh in a Balinese village where few westerners had been. In a Thai monastery I ate the best curries ever, and in Sri Lanka the hottest. I picked olives in Greece and macadamia nuts and feijoas in New Zealand. In the Philippines I was given Malangay (Moringa) soup for wellness.

Always I have been fascinated with food, enjoying creativity with tastes and textures. I never doubted it was a medicine, more conscious of healthy food than many, but not always noticing signs that I should take my understanding further.

In Singapore I picked up the diarrhoea bug Giardia. It kills millions and it tried to kill me. A doctor in Australia said my symptoms were psychological. After six months with wrong diagnoses I was in serious trouble. In desperation I flew home and had more tests in Oxford. They found the bug, gave me the drug and cured me in three weeks. I was not my former super-fit self, but life continued.

In New Zealand a year later I was shopping for whatever vitamin or mineral might make me feel better, and I overheard someone talking about nutrition. I had to speak to him. He was John Carter, a well-loved New Zealand teacher of naturopathy. He put me on an alkaline diet, muscle-tested me for supplements, took me off wheat, sugar and dairy, and became a dear friend.

Looking back, it is hard to understand why I did not stick to alkaline foods and food combining permanently after I had got so much better, but over time I let things slip. I gave up food combining in the hurly burly of getting family food on the table.

I wrote vegetarian recipes for a holistic health magazine and taught Indian vegetarian cookery. At eight, my daughter decided to be completely vegetarian and it was easier for me to follow suit. I went on avoiding sugar, wheat, and pasteurised cow's milk. Interestingly, when we had raw milk from meadow-fed cows it did not upset my system.

In my daughter's teens I gave in and bought her white pasta. When her friends visited she persuaded me to buy pizza because mine were too embarrassingly 'brown'. Some of her friends joked that I was a witch because I had nettles hanging up to dry for tea, and rows of glass jars full of alien foods. They used to dare each other to try things from our fridge.

Now she has found her own strong identity and eats in very healthy ways, but perhaps I am not the only mother who knows how it is wrestling with feeling like an oddity for feeding my family in a natural and healthy way.

Always experimenting and creating, I got a grain grinder and a bread maker. We came home to fresh bread made with rice, barley, oats and rye.

I created an organic cookery course in the Steiner school where I taught. My students cooked everything from scratch and served up meals for teachers and friends at tables set with flowers and napkins. Families eat together less often now and the art of mealtime conversation had to be learned. They chose the dishes and sourced organic ingredients. I took them to an organic farm where they learned about manure and soil, harvested and winnowed oats, hand-milked cows and made butter.

The raw food movement is expanding rapidly and who knows what will be taught in the enlightened schools of the future.

With relatively good eating habits, more knowledge than most people I knew and plenty of fresh greens on my plate, why was I not in perfect health?

Compared to many my age I was very well – no cancer, diabetes, heart disease, obesity or other major problems. But by my late fifties I was exhausted. A gap was growing between what I wanted to do and the energy to do it. I was not Superwoman. Reading books on the sofa appealed more than having an interesting active life.

At the end of 2007 I discovered raw chocolate in Brighton. I loved it and felt full of energy. Online it was heralded as a super-super food, with every micronutrient on the planet. I am grateful it headed me in my raw direction, but not grateful for the caffeine. No wonder I buzzed around feeling wonderful, temporarily.

I bought a kilo of 'cacao liquor', a slab of unsweetened raw dark chocolate. With it I invented divine chocolate treats and imagined becoming a raw chocolatier. Raw chocolate became a daily necessity and my nerves frayed. I had more energy, but it was a roller coaster. I did not have reliable steady energy.

On one prefer-the-sofa evening I read someone saying they would go to the Hippocrates Health Institute in Florida if they were seriously ill. I was not ill but I was curious. I had a vision of a holiday in warm, natural surroundings with good company and healthy food. Perhaps Edinburgh in January breeds such thoughts!

I went online and read the whole Hippocrates site. Next morning, at half past four, I was sitting upright, knowing I had to go to Hippocrates for the full nine weeks Life Transformation Programme and Health Educator Programme.

Things flowed remarkably easily as I was given one of the two last places on the course. I rearranged my work, booked flights and accommodation, and found cat-sitters. Two weeks later, Valentine's Day 2008, I was on the plane.

Hippocrates was nine weeks of fresh wheatgrass, nutritious green juices and living plant food buffets, colonics, lectures, other therapies and emotional work that all helped me to resolve old physical and emotional issues. I learned from delightful fellow guests and students who were doing so much to heal themselves and to live in positive ways. I walked, lounged in hot pools and did exercise classes. I watched racoon families, bright flocks of birds, and turtles slowly paddling around the lake.

While in Florida I was lucky enough to visit several raw food restaurants, to go to raw preparation classes and to attend a raw meal hosted by the raw food writer and restaurant owner Juliano. All this was exquisite new raw fun for my 'inner gourmet', and I hope the future holds more. It was 'recreational food' though, an occasional raw distraction from the living food buffets and juices at the Hippocrates Health institute that were bringing up my levels of reliable energy and wellbeing.

Sometimes I felt dreadful, physically and emotionally, as my body did the major detox it had not been able to do for years. It did not feel like normal illness or the pain from injury. I knew what those were like from intestinal illness and a chronically painful neck injury. These times were more transitory, and in between I felt better and better. I was achieving a much higher level of wellness.

My digestion improved. I sorted out dental issues. My sight improved, and my glasses prescription has hardly changed since. My neck improved. The big change, which was what motivated me to go to Hippocrates, was more energy.

One day at Hippocrates, after a few weeks entirely on raw and living food, a friend saw me striding purposefully along a path through subtropical vegetation and called out, 'You've got as much energy as a teenager!' It was true. I was not even thinking about my body. I was getting on with life, being comfortable in myself, with steady energy and without a single ailment or twinge. I appreciated her telling me that because it helped me to identify a new benchmark of wellness. When you are nearly sixty it is pleasing to be told you are as energetic as a teenager.

Wellness does not feel a particular way, but is about getting on with being me, with less aches, pains, stiffness, ailments, and tiredness. I have had many layers of detoxing to do, physical and emotional, and that process is continuing.

It has been harder to stay well when falling to the side of the raw trail. When travelling in Kenya and Uganda we ate in situations where it would have been foolhardy to eat uncooked food. I did have various raw green powders, super foods and supplements, but still I was more sluggish and had to deal with twinges and tummy 'collywobbles'.

Since studying at Hippocrates, I have had the joy of being back there, informally teaching on the Health Educator Programme, and writing and researching for my book on Wellness.

On the same journey to America I visited the Tree of Life Rejuvenation Centre near the dear little fantasy time-warp cowboy town of Patagonia, Arizona. I went to interview Gabriel and Shanti Cousens for the Wellness book and found myself at a Hindu meditation, an American Indian blanket-giving ceremony, watching humming birds and walking a Celtic labyrinth made of pebbles on the hot, dry grassland. Their raw and living food meals are memorably good, and it was a treat to experience this way of eating flourishing and growing in such a different setting.

I joined a raw potluck group in Glasgow, started one in Edinburgh and visited one in Stirling. I very much enjoyed being in a changing circle of raw food enthusiasts and eating all our lovingly prepared food. I was featured on *The Hour* on Scottish Television, taking along my raw food for the Glaswegian pop star, Lulu. The video of the programme is on my website. I was invited to enter the national *Britain's Best Dish* TV competition with their first ever raw dish, a **Raspberry and Hazelnut**

Cream Tart, and got into the first round. I gave various talks and workshops at home and around Scotland, and co-hosted a raw food event for Dr Brian Clement in Glasgow.

When out, I sometimes eat conventional food for social reasons, and for pleasure. At Burns' night suppers in Edinburgh the central dish and ceremonial focus is a haggis, piped in by bagpipes, praised in Robbie Burn's verse ('chieftain o' the puddin' clan', and all that) and stabbed with a knife from the performer's sock. I was not about to ask for a salad. I had the vegan version but succumbed to Drambuie mousse. It was delicious, but did my cold stay around because of the sugar and milk?

I love Southern Indian food, and if I want the tastes of my favourite Masala Dhosa (filled rice and lentil pancake), I mix Southern Indian spices into raw vegetables. I dehydrate them, wrap them in soft lettuce leaves and serve them with raw chutney and blended raw curry sauce. It is not identical to the traditional dish, but in a way it is more wonderful.

Unless you are very fixed in your tastes, good raw food is good on its own terms. You do not hanker for the cooked food that inspired it when you are busy eating a plate of delicious satisfying raw food. Sometimes I make dehydrated nut sausages and sweet red pepper ketchup for fun and to impress. I did it for the Scottish Herald newspaper. It is not necessary to make and eat that kind of dish, but it may help with staying on track for optimum wellness.

Preparing new dishes is a hobby that satisfies my artistic, creative side. Deciding to write my recipes into a book was a good step that took me on a long journey of inventing, tasting, sharing and testing.

I still feel what I do is cooking because I create meals, but now I know how to make even nicer ones with more nourishment. The food is not heated, but the kitchen still feels like a crucible for transmuting raw ingredients into wonderful meals.

Raw and living food seems to have weighted my system differently so that it rights itself. If I veer into cooked food my taste buds and appetite quickly bring me back to simple raw plant food. So does will power! Knowing I can stay at my benchmark of wellness, I would hardly to settle for less.

What does the future hold? I imagine these recipes rippling out, bringing joy and improved quality of life bringing joy and improved quality of life to many people. I will go on writing, coaching, speaking, teaching and letting life unfold in wonderful ways, knowing that with healthy food as a foundation I can look forward to many happy and productive years.

Please do let me know how the recipes contribute to your food stories by emailing me at judy@judy-barber.com.

In case you want more, I will keep writing down my recipes as I dream them up and collect them for another book. You might find some on my blog too, www.judy-barber.com and www.goodrawfoodrecipes.com and more photos.

Wishing you well and happy

Judy

Index of Recipes

294

Good Resources

Good Books

LIFE FORCE, SUPPLEMENTS EXPOSED, LIVING FOODS FOR OPTIMUM HEALTH, LONGEVITY and other books by **Dr Brian Clement.** Top of my list. Do read at least the first two.

HEALTHY CUISINE **Dr Anna Maria Clement** and **Chef Kelly Serbonich.** Good kitchen information and Hippocrates friendly – recipes.

RAW FOOD WORKS, Leading Experts Explain Why. **Diana Store.** Important overview of cutting edge raw and living food and wellness knowledge.

BE YOUR OWN DOCTOR **Dr Ann Wigmore.** Originated the use of wheatgrass and founded the Hippocrates Health Institute.

CONSCIOUS EATING **Dr Gabriel Cousens.** Tree of Life Rejuvenation Centre www.treeoflife.nu Encyclopedic raw health knowledge and good recipes.

SURVIVAL IN THE 21st CENTURY **Viktoras Kulvinskas.** Good raw and living classic, Hippocrates Health Institute founder, www.viktoras.org

WHEATGRASS, Nature's Finest Medicine **Steve Meyerowitz**. A complete guide to using grasses to revitalise your health.

RAW, The UNcook Book, **Juliano,** raw restaurateur. A colourful, imaginative inspiring raw recipe book – keep an eye on your food combinations.

FOOD WISE, **Wendy Cook.** A sound approach to natural nutritional knowledge, inspired by the work of Rudolf Steiner.

THE CHINA STUDY, **Colin Campbell.** The most comprehensive study of nutrition every conducted, with crucially important implications for diet and health.

THE WORLD PEACE DIET, **Will Tuttle, PhD.** A well-research exploration of the importance of food in personal, societal and environmental change.

FOOD FOR FREE, **Richard Mabey.** Classic illustrated wild food foraging manual.

ME RAW YOU COOKED, **Emma and Rod Macdougall.** Personal exploration of food dynamics for a couple.

TOAST, The Story of a Boy's Hunger, **Nigel Slater.** Moving and entertaining autobiography that illustrates how deeply food and culture affect us.

Good people, events and eating out, UK

ME, **Judy Barber** Hippocrates Health Educator, Living Food and Personal/Professional Coaching, Consultancy, Workshops, Classes, Speaker, NLP, World Cafes, +44-1453756758, www.judy-barber.com and www.goodrawfoodrecipes.com

LIVING FOODS FOR HEALTH **Jill Swyers** Hippocrates Health Educator 16+ years experience, naturopathy, consultancy, speaking, workshops, retreats, +44-2088707041 UK/Portugal, www.jillswyers.com

Wild Food Forager **Rupert Burdock** with whole forests and meadows of knowledge 01453 767553 Stroud Shambles Market, Saturdays.

List of places to eat out on raw food, and other resources, www.funkyraw.com

Brian Clement speaking in the UK: www.fresh-network.com and www.ultimatehealthevents.com

Good Health Spas/Places to Learn

Hippocrates Health Institute, Florida www.hippocratesinst.org

Contact Judy for complimentary support if interested.

Tree of Life Rejuvenation Centre, Arizona www.treeoflife.nu

Good Ingredients online – UK

Quality organic wheatgrass, sunflower greens, snowpea greens, and a variety of sprouts delivered fresh, grains, seeds (with helpful growing instruction sheets) and equipment, **Aconbury Sprouts**, www.wheatgrass-uk.com

Mila, particularly helpful blend of microscopically cut chia seed varieties, http://www.lifemax.net/judybarber/

Pure stevia extract, 'Now' brand, organic, and sauerkraut/kim chi crocks www.ebay.co.uk

HHI-endorsed Lifegive supplements, magazine, raw coconut water, algae including raw frozen bluegreen algae, many helpful foods www.freshnetwork.com

Raw oats, seaweed noodles, soft dulse sea vegetable, algae, many other helpful and treat raw foods www.rawliving.eu

Sun Warrior raw sprouted rice protein powder and HHI-endorsed *Lifegive supplements* www.aggressivehealth.co.uk

Good Equipment online – UK

Juicers, Blenders, Excalibur dehydrators, nut milk bags, water purifiers www.wholisticresearch.com

Juicers, Angel juicer, blenders and other equipment www.juiceland.co.uk

Raw networks

Local raw potluck groups Look for them on www.meetup.com and www.facebook.com, or start one

Give it to me Raw international raw food and holistic living network, www.giveittomeraw.com

Raw in UK raw food forum, www.rawinuk.co.uk

UK Raw food network raw food forum, www.ukrawfoodnetwork.co.uk

Good Resources – USA

Hippocrates Health Institute, Florida, *Lifegive Supplements, books, dvds etc.* www.hippocratesinst.org

Quality wheatgrass, sunflower/snowpea/buckwheat greens, sprouts, seeds, equipment, books and supplies delivered www.gotsprouts.com

Raw food books /vegan books / Living Foods books www.rawplanet.com

Top quality superfood powders www.healthforce.com

Bluegreen algae www.e3live.com

Organic food vitamins www.thesynergycompany.com

About the Author

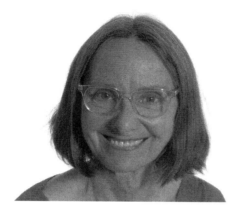

When Judy made her first unsupervised cake at age three, and it was good, they probably realised food would be an important part of her life. It certainly has been. In childhood she roamed the fields for blackberries for jam and sorrel for soup. At school she loved her cookery lessons and often took over the kitchen at home.

Since then, Judy Barber has eaten her way around thirty countries and embraced all kinds of cuisines, including macrobiotics and organic, whole food, vegetarian cookery. She has written recipes for the New Zealand *Whole Health* magazine, taught Indian vegetarian cookery and taught organic cookery at the Edinburgh Rudolf Steiner School. She has also brought up a vegetarian daughter.

On Valentine's Day 2008, Judy landed in Florida and spent nine weeks at the world famous health spa, the Hippocrates Health Institute, where she learned all about delicious raw and living foods and gained her certificate as a Hippocrates Health Educator. She achieved a new benchmark of wellness for herself. Since then Judy has not looked back and she gives presentations, workshops and individual support on food and wellness, as well as creating raw recipes. Judy offers complimentary support for people seriously considering visiting the Hippocrates Health Institute and offers coaching/mentoring before and after your visit.

Meanwhile, Judy continues to weave NLP, Clean Facilitation, Coaching, Social Artistry and World Cafes into her Personal and Professional Development work. She works happily in all these realms and loves combining them with food and wellness topics.

She is the author of *Good Question! The Art of Asking Questions to Bring about Positive Change* and her upcoming book on wellness, which embraces both the emotional and physical aspects of wellness, including what we eat.

Her websites are www.judy-barber.com and www.goodrawfoodrecipes.com
Contact Judy at judy@judy-barber.com

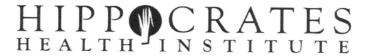

HIPP◉CRATES
HEALTH INSTITUTE

www.HippocratesInstitute.org

For over half a century, the Hippocrates Health Institute has helped people prevent and reverse disease as well as the premature aging process.

Guests from all over the world travel to West Palm Beach, Florida, to benefit from health and nutritional counselling, non-invasive remedial and youth-enhancing therapies, state of the art spa services, inspiring talks on life principles and a tantalizing daily buffet of enzyme-rich, organic meals. Health-minded people attend the Hippocrates Life Transformation Programme in equal numbers to those who visit to reverse disease.

For those who are new to the living food lifestyle, Hippocrates makes this a comfortable transition. The medical team and professional care servers support guests as they transform their lives in an encouraging environment, along with others who are recovering from similar challenges.

HHI alumni are people from all walks of life who have benefited from the institute's blueprint. They share stories of recovery that are considered miraculous by some, but are actually quite typical of people who have embraced the Hippocrates lifestyle. After graduating, alumni are afforded the privilege of periodic, lifelong, written counsel.

For more information Call (561) 471-8876 ext. 2177 and visit our website www.hippocratesinstitute.com

Hippocrates Health Institute (Florida)
www.hippocratesinst.org
1 – 877 – 582 – 5850 – toll free within USA
+ 1 561 471 8876 – ext: 171

Also by this author...

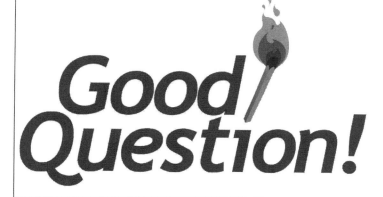

"A treasure-trove of pearls from inspirational coaches and experts in many fields of personal and business development, Good Question! helps you answer, and guide others to answer, so many of life's biggest questions."

Amanda Wise, www.wiselifecoaching.com

Good Question!

the art of asking questions to bring about positive change

Judy Barber

Richard Wilkins, Mark Forster, Coen de Groot, David Ure, Deepak Lodhia, Ewemade Orobator, David Hyner, Gary Outrageous, Julie French, Richard Tod, Tessa Lovemore, George Metcalfe, Martin Haworth, Steve Halls, Gérard Jakimavicius, Joe Armstrong, Wendy Sullivan, Sanjay Shah, Tony Burgess, Jamie Smart, Debbie Jenkins, Gerard O'Donovan, Jesvir Mahil, Jean Houston, Chris Howe, Lisa Wynn, Babu Shah, Aboodi Shabi, Lourdes Callen

Find out more at www.judy-barber.com and
www.goodrawfoodrecipes.com

14184421R00175

Printed in Great Britain
by Amazon.co.uk, Ltd.,
Marston Gate.